*Biologically Informed
Psychotherapy
for Depression*

Biologically Informed Psychotherapy for Depression

STEPHEN R. SHUCHTER, M.D.
NANCY DOWNS, M.D.
SIDNEY ZISOOK, M.D.

THE GUILFORD PRESS
New York   London

Last digit is print number: 9   8   7   6   5   4   3   2   1

Library of Congress Cataloging-in-Publication Data

Shuchter, Stephen R.
    Biologically informed psychotherapy for depression / Stephen R.
Shuchter, Nancy Downs, Sidney Zisook.
        p.   cm.
    Includes bibliographical references and index.
    ISBN 1-57230-069-8
    1.   Depression, Mental—Treatment.   2. Depression, Mental—
Pathophysiology.   3. Psychotherapy.   I. Downs, Nancy.   II. Zisook,
Sidney, 1943–   .   III. Title.
    [DNLM: 1. Depression—therapy.   2. Psychotherapy—methods.
3. Models, Biological.   WM 171S562b 1996]
RC537.S387 1996
616.85'2706—dc20
DNLM/DLC
for Library of Congress   96-4858
                                                                                 CIP

Preface

The purpose of this book is to present clinicians of all disciplines with an integrated approach to the psychotherapy of patients with depressive disorders that incorporates modern biological knowledge pertaining to these disorders. We call this approach "biologically informed psychotherapy for depression."

Psychodynamic theory has dominated clinical training in psychotherapy by mental health professionals since the 1950s. At that time, the mental health field knew little about the role of neurobiology in the pathogenesis of psychiatric disorders or about the profound impact that various psychotropic medications would have on their course and prognosis. As a result of technical advances and the growth of scientific methodology during the remainder of the 20th century, we have seen an explosion of information about the biological nature of many of the more common and disabling disturbances of brain function, including schizophrenic disorders, bipolar and other affective disorders, and, more recently, the anxiety disorders, alcoholism, and eating disorders. From studies of phenomenology, epidemiology, genetics, neurophysiology, brain structural and functional anatomy, basic cellular mechanisms, and psychopharmacology, there has emerged an enormous body of biobehavioral knowledge about these disorders.

Most of this body of knowledge did not exist when psychological theories regarding the nature and treatment of mood disturbances were developed. Moreover, biological concepts and knowledge have not greatly influenced the evolution of psychotherapeutic treatment approaches. Nor has there been much clarification of how psychodynamic and other primarily psychological approaches interact with biological approaches, despite the fact that clinical practitioners struggle regularly with their interaction. The frequently asked question "Is depression biological or psychological?" reflects thinking that has not yet integrated psychodynamic understanding with biological knowledge. Thus, patient care often remains fragmented, rather than incorporating a full and comprehensive understanding and integration of the psychological and biological knowledge bases.

Parallel to these advances in understanding the biological basis and treatment for many mental disorders, there has been an expanding literature on the empirical study of psychosocial, cognitive, and behavioral approaches to treating these disorders, again with a preponderance of evidence demonstrating the efficacy of such approaches in treating specific disorders. With empirical support for these treatments, there has been an increasing "eclectification" of treatment for patients suffering from major psychiatric disorders, with therapists of many disciplines—psychiatry, psychology, social work, nursing, and marriage and family counseling—employing theoretical frameworks and practical techniques that will be helpful to their patients. As more and more studies demonstrate the additive effects of combining medical with psychological, cognitive, and behavioral therapies, and as mental health care delivery systems investigate the most cost-effective approaches to treatment, there has been an increasing tendency toward compartmentalization by discipline: Nonphysician psychotherapists provide some form of ongoing exploratory, supportive, cognitive, or behavioral treatment, whereas psychiatrists or other primary care physicians provide psychopharmacological interventions. In some circumstances, there are "teams" working within an organized system, and treatment is formally coordinated by these teams. In others, independent medical and nonmedical practitioners communicate about their work with the same patients. In still other settings, clinicians may have little knowledge about the work being done by their cotherapists. Finally, some psychiatrists provide both psychotherapeutic and psychopharmacological treatment to their patients.

We have spent the past 20 years practicing, consulting, and teaching in large, "modern" university training centers in "enlightened" communities. We have found that the majority of clinicians approach patients with a psychodynamically based, eclectic patchwork of helpful therapies, but that few clinicians provide truly integrated treatment of psychiatric disorders. By "integrated treatment," we mean not only the artful application of the best scientifically based pharmacological knowledge, but also a psychotherapeutic approach that attends to a dynamic understanding of the pathology being treated. Biologically informed psychotherapy for depression attempts to achieve this integration.

Chapter 1 begins with an overview of historical approaches to the treatment of depression and the evolution of scientific understanding of how the brain works. There is a review of each of the major biological models of depression, including neurotransmitter, neuroreceptor regulatory, and neurohumoral hypotheses; theories of circadian rhythm abnormalities, sleep disturbances, and kindling with behavioral sensitization; and genetic and anatomic hypotheses. Also included is an overview of psychopharmacological and alternative treatments for depression. Chapter 2 examines some of the fundamental assumptions about psychopathology that are contained in both psychodynamic and biological models. Although there are some areas of overlap, the inconsistencies and distinctly contradictory views are underscored.

Chapter 3 reviews the primary symptoms of depression and presents the DSM-IV criteria for the two primary depressive conditions. Chapter 4 elaborates the "language" of depression—the myriad ways in which depression is elaborated into intrapsychic, interpersonal, and functional phenomena that tend to undermine a depressed person's capacity to live in the world. These manifestations of depression represent the greatest threat to the individual and become a central focus for continued evaluation and treatment.

Chapter 5 describes the general and specific approaches to treating depression that evolve from the perspective presented in the earlier chapters. Although we borrow heavily from educational, behavioral, cognitive, dynamic, interpersonal, family, and supportive therapies, we orient our approach around a central concept and its corollaries. The fact is that depression is an *autonomous* disorder: It has a life of its own, relatively independent of its contributing factors. Consequently, treatment is focused on its control or management and on the limitation of its potential effects. This requires a thorough understanding of and "battle" against the sometimes insidious and sometimes blatant forces of regression, which are the *effects of* and *not the causes of* depression. This pivotal and perhaps controversial view leads to the reexamination of many long-held tenets in the psychotherapeutic treatment of depression, including an indictment of some traditional approaches as potentially harmful.

Chapter 6 outlines the structure of treatment planning, design, and conduct of the psychotherapy. Chapter 7 presents a comparison of biologically informed psychotherapy with the other major researched psychotherapies for depression: cognitive-behavioral therapy, interpersonal psychotherapy, and short-term dynamic psychotherapy. Chapter 8 offers an overview of six patients' treatment with biologically informed psychotherapy for depression. Finally, Chapter 9 offers a glimpse of how the principles of biologically informed psychotherapy for depression may be applied to various other states of regression, including anxiety disorders, mania, and schizophrenia.

In presenting this approach to the treatment of depression, and its application to other symptomatic disorders, it is our intent to introduce a way of thinking about psychotherapeutic processes based on assumptions about the biological underpinnings of these disorders. Two warn-ings are in order, however. The first is that many facets of psychopathol-ogy have yet to be revealed. We believe we have good guesses that have been derived from scientific inquiry, but the views that Freud and others once fervently held have had to be modified in the light of present-day knowledge; it is possible, or even likely, that current views will likewise soon be seen as naive. In this case, further revision of our "best guesses" and their implications for future psychotherapeutics will be important. This brings us to the second warning: This book is not a prescription for treatment but a set of guidelines, which, even if they have some valid-ity, still require continued intellectual work and artful application to each patient's unique life and circumstances.

STEPHEN R. SHUCHTER
NANCY DOWNS
SIDNEY ZISOOK

Contents

*Biologically Informed
Psychotherapy
for Depression*

· 1 ·

Biological Models of Depressive Disorders

This chapter takes the reader on a brief tour of the evolution of biological concepts and biological research in depression. It first provides a historical overview, and then reviews the major hypotheses regarding the biology of depression. These include the following:

1. Genetic hypotheses
2. Neurotransmitter hypotheses
3. Neuroreceptor regulation hypotheses
4. Neuroendocrine hypotheses
5. Circadian rhythm and sleep disturbances hypotheses
6. Kindling and behavioral sensitization hypotheses

The chapter also includes a review of the major psychopharmacological treatments, and concludes by noting the movement toward a synthesis of the various hypotheses.

HISTORICAL OVERVIEW

Although depression has been described in the literature of all cultures through antiquity, the first formal notions of its biological substrates were contained in the Hippocratic theory of melancholia (literally, "black bile"). This view of depression as a consequence of internal, physically toxic processes that have profound effects on the whole of the victim's existence is closer to the current biological understanding of depression than any other perspective that has existed in the intervening 2,000 years.

The scientific study of depression began about 100 years ago, but made limited progress until the serendipitous discovery of antidepressant medications in the early 1950s. At that time, tubercular patients

1

treated with the antitubercular drug iproniazid, a monoamine oxidase inhibitor (MAOI), showed dramatic responses to the medication in terms of mood changes. Some patients found that coexisting depressions improved, whereas other patients developed mania. The development of the tricyclic antidepressant (TCA) medications amitriptyline (another serendipitous discovery in the search for a more effective form of chlorpromazine) and imipramine broadened a repertoire of biological treatments that had previously been limited to insulin shock and electroconvulsive therapy (ECT), as well as the relatively ineffective stimulants and analgesic–sedatives.

From these beginnings has evolved an extraordinary body of clinical and basic research into the mechanisms of brain functions in depression and the efficacy of biological treatments for depression. Parallel and essential developments in this scientific evolution have been the systematic observation and classification of clinical phenomena (derived from the Kraepelinian school of psychiatry) and their transformation into reliable and reproducible diagnostic tools; the increasing sophistication of research methodology, including computer and statistical approaches that have enhanced the use of available data; the development of clinical rating scales to assess psychopathology and fine-tune clinical outcome studies; and a broadened base of empiricism as the most acceptable road to knowledge in all modern societies. The most recent two decades have seen the development of various means of visualizing the brain and its functioning: magnetic resonance imaging (MRI), computed tomography (CT), positron emission tomography (PET), and single photon emission computed tomography (SPECT).

The remainder of this chapter examines some of the many biological models that have evolved in our current understanding of depression, and also provides a review of psychopharmacology.

GENETIC HYPOTHESES

The first twin study of affective disorders (Luxenburger, 1930) demonstrated that relatives of persons with affective disorders had an increased risk of developing such disorders. For the next 50 years numerous studies, with increasing methodological sophistication, replicated and expanded the thesis that there exists a spectrum of inherited disorders that includes unipolar depressive disorders, bipolar disorders, and cyclothymic disorder, as well as schizoaffective disorders, anorexia nervosa, and suicide. Unipolar depressive disorders appear to be a more heterogeneous group than bipolar disorders in terms of heritable conditions, including a separate form that may be cotransmitted with alcoholism (Goldin & Gershon, 1983).

The strongest evidence for heritability has come from twin studies, which have repeatedly demonstrated the greater concordance rate of affective illness among monozygotic (MZ) than among dizygotic (DZ) twins. The Danish twin studies (Bertelsen et al., 1977), epidemiologically the soundest, found a concordance rate of 67% among 55 MZ pairs and 20% among 52 DZ pairs. The concordance rate for bipolar disorders was 79% among MZ pairs, compared to 54% for unipolar depression among MZ pairs; this suggests some stronger genetic loading for bipolar than for unipolar disorders. However, the concordance among DZ pairs was similar for bipolar and unipolar disorders (24% and 19%, respectively). Variable concordance rates were determined for different forms and severities of affective disorder among MZ pairs:

Bipolar I (depression and clinical mania)	80%
Bipolar II (depression and clinical hypomania)	78%
Unipolar (<3 episodes of depression)	59%
Unipolar (<3 episodes of depression)	33% (to time of study)

Adoption studies have played an important role in determining the importance of prenatal and perinatal factors in the subsequent development of an affective disorder. The basic design of such studies is to determine the rate of illness of high-risk offspring (children born to parents with affective illness) who are adopted out of their biological parents' homes at birth and reared in other settings. Table 1.1 compares the rates of affective disorder obtained in one such study (Mendlewicz & Rainer, 1977) for the biological and adoptive parents of affectively disordered adoptees, the biological parents of nonadopted children with affective disorder, and both the biological and adoptive parents of normal adoptees. In other adoption studies, biological relatives of disordered adoptees were found to be substantially more likely to commit suicide than their adoptive relatives, or than either the biological or adoptive relatives of normal adoptees (Schulsinger et al., 1979; Kety, 1979).

Family studies have repeatedly demonstrated that bipolar disorders

TABLE 1.1. Rates of Affective Disorder in One Adoption Study

	Biological parents	Adoptive parents
Affectively disordered adoptees	31%	12%
Nonadopted affectively disordered children	26%	—
Normal adoptees	2%	9%

Note. Data from Mendlewicz & Rainer (1977).

are more "penetrable" than unipolar disorders. That is, unipolar histories are more common in the offspring and extended families of bipolar patients than vice versa (Gershon et al., 1987). The penetrability of affective disorders also appears in studies of the time of onset of such illnesses: The earlier the onset of an affective disorder, the greater the risk of illness in relatives of the proband (Gershon et al., 1976).

During the past decade, new strategies reflecting advances in scientific technology have evolved for the study of genetic transmission of affective illness. Among these new strategies is the correlation of diagnostic data among patients and their relatives with chromosomal linkage markers or pathophysiological vulnerability markers (Egeland et al., 1987; Baron et al., 1987). Genetic research in psychiatry has begun to focus on the identification and characterization of events at a single gene locus. Much of this research has focused specifically on the X chromosome and chromosome 11 in relation to affective disorders.

The hypothesis that manic–depressive illness is transmitted by a gene on the X chromosome was suggested in 1935 by Rosanoff et al. The first evidence for this hypothesis was reported over 30 years later (Winokur et al., 1969). In Winokur's study, two lines of data suggested that manic–depressive illness was X-linked: (1) Family study data showed an increased risk of transmission to females and an absence of transmission from male to male; and (2) there were two bipolar pedigrees in which bipolar disorder was associated with color-blindness, an X-linked trait. Subsequent studies have correlated manic–depressive illness with such X-linked markers as blood groups (Mendlewicz & Fleiss, 1974) and a deficiency of an enzyme, glucose-6-phosphate dehydrogenase (Mendlewicz et al., 1980). Numerous family pedigrees with these X linkages continue to be studied, including a cohort of Sephardic Jewish families; all are suggestive of at least a subtype of manic–depressive illness with X-linked inheritance (Baron et al., 1987).

In order to examine a relatively homogeneous population with sufficiently large pedigrees that are "uncontaminated" by marriage, a group from the National Institute of Mental Health (NIMH) studied the Amish population, a group that is fairly isolated and relatively "pure" (Egeland et al., 1987). One Amish pedigree suggested an autosomal dominant transmission and the linkage of both bipolar and unipolar illness to a section of chromosome 11 (Egeland et al., 1987). Other studies of different Amish pedigrees (Detera-Wadleigh et al., 1987) and of three Icelandic pedigrees (Hodgkinson et al., 1987) failed to replicate this finding. Because of the methodological soundness of the first study, it appears that there may be heterogeneity in this disorder, with the first Amish pedigree's form of manic–depressive illness being uncommon in the other populations; or perhaps there is another necessary linkage that was not determined. The elucidation of such genetic markers is now at the fore-front of biological research in psychiatry, both because of its heuristic value and because it is hoped that future technologies such as genetic recombination will offer a definitive "cure" for a devastating illness.

NEUROTRANSMITTER HYPOTHESES

Scientific knowledge of brain function expanded significantly with the discovery and elucidation of the functions of neurotransmitters. "Neuro-transmitters" are chemical substances that are (1) synthesized in a neu-ron (nerve cell), (2) released from a presynaptic terminal, and (3) exert their influence on a receptor neuron. New neurotransmitters continue to be discovered; the earliest to be identified as playing possible roles in affective illness are listed in Table 1.2.

In 1965, Schildkraut presented the catecholamine hypothesis of affective disorders. He postulated that depression is associated with a func-tional deficiency of norepinephrine (NE) in significant synapses in the brain (see Figure 1.1), whereas mania is a product of excessive NE or noradrenergic functions. The evidence for this hypothesis was derived initially from the empirical findings of the efficacy of both MAOIs and TCAs in relieving depression. Each drug appeared to have a different mechanism of action, but both mechanisms were consistent with the cat-echolamine hypothesis. MAOIs seemed to work by preventing the oxida-tive metabolism of NE, thereby increasing its functional availability for neu-ronal transmission. TCAs were thought to be effective by blocking the active metabolic reuptake of NE into presynaptic storage, making NE more available in a relative way by depleting its storage. Further support for the hypothesis came from the observation that 15% of patients treated with reserpine, an antihypertensive that worked through the depletion of peri-pheral (and central) biogenic amines, developed significant depressive symptoms (Schildkraut, 1965; Bunney & Davis, 1965).

TABLE 1.2. "Early" Neurotransmitters Implicated in Affective Disorders

Amino acids	Biogenic amines	Cholinergic agents
Gamma-aminobutyric acid (GABA)	Norepinephrine (NE)	Acetylcholine
Glutamate	Dopamine (DA)	
Glycine	Serotonin (5-HT)	
	Histamine	

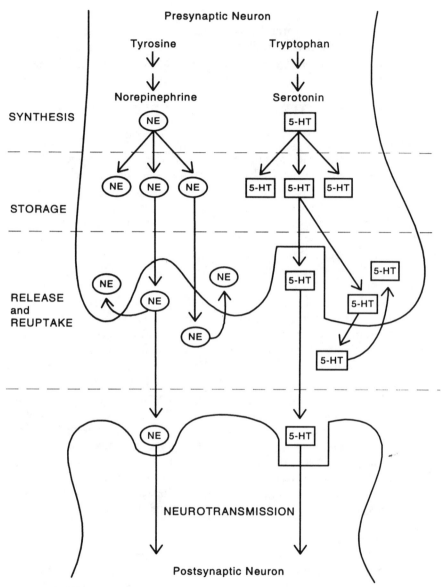

FIGURE 1.1. Noradrenergic and serotonergic neuronal activity.

During the past three decades, exploration of the catecholamine hypothesis has taken several directions. For instance, studies of the brain and cerebrospinal fluid for metabolites of NE have demonstrated elevations in such metabolites (e.g., 3-methoxy-4-hydroxyphenylglycol [MHPG]) in patients with mania (Swann et al., 1987), but rather equivocal finds in depressed patients (Schildkraut, 1965; Schildkraut et al., 1978; Schatzberg et al., 1982). Examinations of the urinary excretion of MHPG have generally, but not consistently, found lower levels in depressed patients and higher levels in manic patients than in normal controls. In another line of research, a finding in suicide victims of an increased number of beta-adrenergic receptors in prefrontal cortical tissue suggested an up-regulation of these postsynaptic receptors because of a reduction in presynaptic NE activity (Mann & Stanley, 1986). Still other studies (Potter et al., 1985; Koslow et al., 1983) have determined that there is a great range of measurable NE activity in depressed patients, raising issues of the heterogeneity of depression, the admixture of anxiety-related phenomena, and the validity of the "pure" catecholamine hypothesis.

Whereas the original catecholamine hypothesis focused on NE dysfunction, a parallel hypothesis has viewed depressive disorders as a consequence of deficient brain serotonin (5-HT) (Coppen et al., 1972). There is much evidence that decreased 5-HT activity can either increase vulnerability to or cause depression. 5-HT is widely distributed in the brain and has many interactions with other neurotransmitters. 5-HT activity has been associated with numerous processes that are dysregulated in depression, including negative mood, sleep disturbances, shortened rapid-eye-movement (REM) latency, disturbed circadian rhythms, abnormal neuroendocrine functions, and sexual abnormalities. 5-HT and its major metabolite, 5-hydroxyindoleacetic acid (5-HIAA), have been found to be depleted both in the brains of suicide victims and in the cerebrospinal fluid of depressed patients (Mann & Stanley, 1986).

The reuptake-blocking effects of both MAOIs and TCAs increase levels of 5-HT (Shopsin et al., 1974). Also, the antidepressant effects of these medications are reversed by the addition of the 5-HT-depleting drug parachlorophenylalamine (Shopsin et al., 1974). The addition of lithium carbonate, which may increase 5-HT production, has been shown to enhance the effectiveness of TCAs in treating depressed patients (DeMontigny et al., 1983). The development during the 1980s and 1990s of selective serotonin reuptake inhibitors (SSRIs), such as fluoxetine, sertraline, paroxetine, and fluvoxamine, has also provided strong evidence in support of the 5-HT hypothesis. These medications demonstrate high degrees of specificity in their capacity to block 5-HT and not NE reuptake.

The research described here is representative of only a small fraction of the thousands of studies that have explored the neurotransmitter hypotheses. However, many studies have obtained equivocal findings or some that are contrary to these hypotheses. Our understanding of the mechanisms of action of antidepressants is challenged by the facts that the inhibition of monoamine reuptake occurs within hours or days, yet clinical benefits may not occur for weeks after treatment begins. There are also a number of agents that are very effective antidepressants but that do not seem to affect 5-HT or NE reuptake or metabolic degradation; these include bupropion and mianserin. Despite their ability to block monoamine reuptake, amphetamines probably are not effective antidepressants. As a consequence of such discrepancies, other models of depression have been explored.

NEURORECEPTOR REGULATION HYPOTHESES

Alternative hypotheses to neurotransmitter dysregulation suggest that depression may represent altered or diminished function at the site of the neuroreceptor on the postsynaptic neuron (see Figure 1.1). It is suggested that the discrepancy between the onset of reuptake inhibition and the therapeutic action of TCAs may be accounted for by changes occurring over time at the receptor site. Charney et al. (1981) have demonstrated decreased serotonergic as well as noradrenergic receptor activity following chronic antidepressant treatment. These findings were not restricted to any particular type of antidepressant, but were generally present with all types, including those that are not typical TCAs and MAOIs (Sulser, 1986; Peroutka & Snyder, 1980).

Adrenergic and serotonergic receptors exist both centrally in the brain and peripherally in other organ systems. Peripheral receptors have been studied by using lymphocytes (Mann et al., 1985) and platelets (Garcia-Sevilla et al., 1981) to define their quantities and such qualities as binding capacities and functional associations. Extrapolation from the findings on these peripheral receptors to central receptors has been warranted by their similarities and their ease of availability, despite our ignorance of the relationship between the two types of receptors. The advantages of studying peripheral blood receptors are that they may reflect systemic changes in receptor functions; they can be observed without affecting any neuronal changes; and clinical changes can be correlated with parallel assays of these receptors. The disadvantage is that the regulation of each type of receptors is likely to be different. Because of the heterogeneity of depression and the variability and overlap of results between depressed patients and controls (Mann et al., 1985; Garcia-Sevilla et al., 1981), such measures have limited value as biological markers.

Other research strategies indicating that affective illness is associated with alterations in neuronal receptor sensitivity are pharmacological challenges in normal volunteers, as well as in patients with depression (but acute and in remission), to probe adrenergic and cholinergic sensitivity.

NEUROENDOCRINE HYPOTHESES

Depressive disorders are characterized by numerous changes in the functioning of hypothalamic centers, which regulate eating, pleasure, sexual drives, circadian rhythms, and the synthesis and release of hypothalamic hormones (Sacher et al., 1970; Carroll et al., 1976; Gold et al., 1988). Depressed patients exhibit inhibited or excessive eating behavior, a loss of pleasure and sexual interest, alterations of the sleep–wake cycle (with either increased or diminished sleep), and diurnal mood changes (Gold et al., 1988). Importantly, neurotransmitters have mediative effects on most endocrine functions.

Cortisol Abnormalities

The hypothalamic–pituitary–adrenal (HPA) axis is the system that mediates the generalized stress response described by Selye (1936, 1950). When homeostasis is threatened, the elements of this connecting system initiate or facilitate the central neural pathways that promote attention, arousal, and aggression, while inhibiting the pathways of such vegetative functions as eating, sexual behavior, and reproduction. Peripheral systems act through catecholamines to raise heart rate and blood pressure, and through glucocorticoids to mobilize fuel for immediate action.

Figure 1.2 shows the mechanisms involved in normal cortisol production. The hypothalamus synthesizes corticotropin-releasing factor (CRF), which initiates the pituitary release of adrenocorticotropic hormone (ACTH). ACTH influences the adrenal release of cortisol, which acts both centrally and peripherally in the stress response system and as an inhibitor of the hypothalamic synthesis of CRF.

In depression, this mechanism goes awry: Hypercortisolism is regularly found, particularly in melancholic forms of depression (Carroll et al., 1976). This finding has been elaborated in many studies of depression that have employed the dexamethasone suppression test (DST). Normal people given a small dose of the synthetic hormone dexametha-

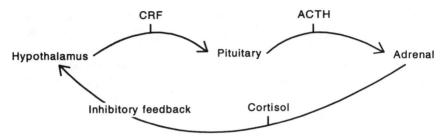

FIGURE 1.2. Mechanisms involved in normal cortisol production.

sone will demonstrate a lowering of plasma cortisol levels. Elevated levels of plasma cortisol following dexamethasone administration have been found in depressed patients. However, this finding has also been seen in patients with mania, dementia, eating disorders, and acute grief, and as a reaction to some medical conditions (Nemeroff, 1989; Shuchter et al., 1986; Gold et al., 1986). Its nonspecificity has disappointed those who hoped that the DST might prove to be a useful diagnostic tool or a means of following treatment response in depression.

Thyroid Abnormalities

The association between depression and both hypothyroidism and hyperthyroidism has been clearly identified in medicine and endocrinology. Figure 1.3 shows the relationships involved in normal thyroid regulation. In recent years, there have been studies demonstrating that "subclinical" hypothyroid conditions can also produce depression. This can occur in patients whose traditional thyroid function tests are considered normal but who demonstrate increases in production of thyroid-stimulating hormone (TSH) or an abnormally blunted TSH response to thyrotropin-releasing hormone (TRH) (Loosen, 1985; Loosen & Prange, 1982). This latter finding is the basis of the TRH test, developed with the hope of its being a specific diagnostic tool for depression. Like the DST, the TRH test has proven to be another nonspecific measure of HPA axis dysregulation, although it still holds some promise for future clinical utility and for research on the pathophysiology of depression.

Melatonin Abnormalities

Another promising area of study in the neuroendocrinology of depression has been the pineal gland's production of the hormone melatonin. This hormone is of particular interest, because its synthesis is almost exclusively under the control of noradrenergic neurotransmission, and thus it has become a marker for NE activity. The pineal gland synthe-

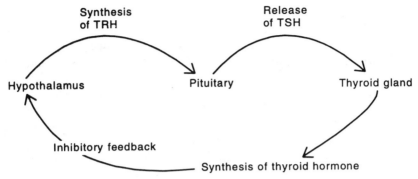

FIGURE 1.3. Mechanisms involved in normal thyroid regulation.

sizes melatonin at night, and this nocturnal synthesis has been found to be diminished in depressed patients (Brown et al., 1985). Exposure of depressed patients to increased sunlight has both ameliorative effects on depressed patients with seasonal affective disorders and melatonin-enhancing effects (Lewy et al., 1987; Wehr et al., 1986). (See "Circadian Rhythm Alterations," below.)

Reproductive Endocrinology

Physicians and psychiatrists have long been aware of the association between reproductive functions in women and specific depressive syndromes. These include postpartum depression, premenstrual dysphoric disorder, and menopause-related depression. Endocrinological changes are clearly associated with both postpartum depression (in which average estrogen and progesterone levels may drop as much as 100-fold from a week before delivery to a week after delivery) and menopausally precipitated depression. By contrast, premenstrual dysphoric disorder has shown no hormonal patterns consistently suggestive of insufficient or excessive amounts of reproductive hormones that might correlate directly with depression. All of these syndromes occur with significantly increased frequency among women with a preexisting mood disturbance. (For a fuller discussion of the syndromes, see Gitlin & Pasnau, 1989.)

CIRCADIAN RHYTHM AND SLEEP
DISTURBANCE HYPOTHESES

Circadian Rhythm Alterations

There is a subset of depressed patients whose disorder may reflect altered circadian rhythms. Circadian (daily) rhythms are responsible for the normal regulation of sleep–wake cycles, patterns of arousal and activity, and the corresponding patterns of hormonal secretions that are both responsible for and reactive to such rhythms. They are influenced by the effects of bright light to which the eye is exposed, but appear to be in the "hard-wiring" for most species. Humans who are totally blind are found to have free-running melatonin and cortisol rhythms with an average circadian period of 24.6 hours, similar to that of humans living in temporal isolation (Aschoff, 1969; Wever, 1979). This inclination toward a "phase delay" is compensated for by the use of external cues and time adjustments for sleep and activity.

Winter depression is a specific example of depression that may be attributable to the desynchronization of different biological functions associated with a phase delay in circadian rhythms. Normally, temperature and cortisol levels are at their nadir in the early morning (2–3 A.M.) and reach their peak at an individual's usual point of awakening, thereby preparing the person for arousal and activity. As the amount of bright light subsides in the winter months, a phase delay can lead to a shift in levels of arousal and wakefulness—the hypersomnia of winter depression (Aschoff, 1969; Wever, 1979; Czeisler et al., 1980; Beersma et al., 1984). Phase delay can also be produced by shift work when sleep is put off to a later time, or by "jet lag" after one has traveled from east to west through several time zones. Each of these circumstances can produce depressive-like states in which time-cued sleep–wake cycles are dissociated and delayed from normal circadian rhythms.

This view is supported by the corollary that circumstances producing a phase *advance* in circadian rhythm seem to have therapeutic benefit for many forms of depression (Wehr et al., 1979). These include increased exposure, particularly in the early morning, to bright light (Lewy et al., 1987; Wehr et al., 1986); sleep deprivation; and west-to-east air travel.

Sleep Disturbances

Electrophysiological studies of sleep have consistently found abnormalities of sleep architecture associated with depression. The most consistent, replicable finding has been "shortened REM latency" (Kupfer & Foster, 1972; Coble et al., 1976; Gillin et al., 1979). Normally, an individual goes through four stages of sleep (stages 1 and 2 are lighter; stages 3 and 4 are deeper) before entering REM sleep. REM sleep is the stage in which dreaming is presumed to occur. It is "paradoxical sleep" in the sense that although pulse, respiration, blood pressure, and brain metabolism are all elevated above the levels found in non-REM sleep or even many waking states, at the same time there is an almost total motor inhibition, with absence of body movements. The amount of time until the first appearance of REM sleep ("REM latency") is normally 90 minutes; REM sleep then occurs every 90–100 minutes and lasts from 10 to 40 minutes each time (the length increases throughout the night), totaling about 25% of sleep time (Gillin et al., 1984).

In depression, REM latency is abbreviated, total REM time is increased, and stages 3 and 4 are diminished. Depressed patients describe having less sleep, more disrupted sleep, and more intense and frequent dreaming. These changes have generally been viewed as manifestations of depression. However, the notion that sleep disturbances may play a more causal role in the development of depression comes from three kinds of data. First, sleep disturbances frequently appear very early in the evolution of a depressive episode. Second, antidepressant medications usually increase stage 3 and stage 4 sleep while diminishing REM time. Finally, sleep deprivation may at least temporarily reverse the effects of depression (Gillin et al., 1984).

KINDLING AND BEHAVIORAL
SENSITIZATION HYPOTHESES

"Kindling" describes an electrophysiological phenomenon that is well described in neurology as it pertains to seizure activity. Following electrical stimulation of brain regions at subdepolarization levels over time, an animal will develop full-blown seizures spontaneously. If this is done early in life, the tendency to produce seizures will often persist. Clinical seizure activity, untreated, will tend to accelerate and become even more severe and spontaneous (Goddard et al., 1969; Pine & Van Oot, 1975; Janowsky et al., 1980).

Several features of the natural history of affective illness are addressed in the kindling model (Post et al., 1981; Cutter & Post, 1982). These include the following:

1. Predisposition toward depression by early life stressors
2. An acceleration in frequency of depression over time
3. Worsening of episodes over time
4. The rapidity with which subsequent episodes intensify in severity
5. Evolution of spontaneity and autonomy of episodes, with a consequent tendency toward chronicity

A parallel process is that of behavioral sensitization, wherein are seen long-term changes in the responsivity of the central nervous system. Changes in neurological excitability can be seen through sensitization to the behavioral effects of psychomotor stimulants after repeated, intermittent application (Post et al., 1981; Shuster et al., 1977; Post, 1980). Furthermore, experimental stress can reduce the threshold of stimulant-induced sensitization, and repeated stresses alone can produce such effects (MacLennan & Maier, 1983). The "learned helplessness" model of depression (Seligman, 1975) is based on experiments in which inescapable shocks were provided to rats; these produced progressive increases in behavioral and neurochemical abnormalities (Cassens et al., 1980).

The kindling and behavioral sensitization models hold that early, painful experiences of loss may sensitize persons who subsequently develop depression, such that their vulnerability to such states persists and worsens with time, resulting in recurrent dysphoria even when the original form of the stimulus is gone. Evidence supporting these hypotheses include the data that the anticonvulsant carbamazepine, which inhibits kindled seizures, and lithium, which can block behavioral sensitization, both have prophylactic effects in treating manic–depressive illness (Ballenger & Post, 1969; Wada et al., 1976; Post, 1987; Post et al., 1981).

ANATOMIC SUBSTRATES

A landmark discovery in the behavioral neurosciences occurred in 1963, when it was found that Parkinson's disease was associated with the loss of dopamine (DA) activity in the basal ganglia due to the degeneration of DA-producing cells (Hornykiewicz, 1963). This was the first clear demonstration that a specific neurotransmitter deficiency was related to a specific behavioral syndrome. Subsequent neurotransmitter hypotheses, as well as psychopharmacological interventions, have extended the view that psychopathological states are products of increases or decreases in specific neurotransmitters (Goodwin & Jamison, 1984). Studies of brain structure using MRI have shown ventricular enlargement with focal volume loss in the temporal lobes of the brains of schizophrenic patients (Weinberger et al., 1980; Andreasen et al., 1990). Fewer studies have been done on patients with affective disorders (Jeste et al., 1988), and the findings have been inconsistent. CT studies have noted ventricular enlargement, cortical atrophy, and cerebellar atrophy in affective patients, but these have not been confirmed (Nasrallah et al., 1989). Contrast studies have demonstrated focal abnormalities (Bench et al., 1992; George et al., 1993). MRI studies of patients with unipolar and bipolar disorders have suggested ventricular enlargement and subcortical abnormalities, including diminished size of the caudate nucleus (Nasrallah et al., 1989). The notion that there may be brain structural abnormalities in depressive disorders may suggest an explanation for alterations in neurotransmitter availability.

An alternative model for understanding the relationship between neurotransmission and psychopathological states involves an integrative model of neural circuitry that looks at normal functioning of the circuitry and hypothesizes how dysfunction in a single aspect of such a system could contribute to behavioral abnormalities occurring in different disease processes (Swerdlow & Koob, 1987). Figure 1.4 is a schematic representation of normal limbic circuitry in the brain, depicting afferent and efferent connections among a number of limbic structures: the cortex, the striatum, the pallidum, and the thalamus. It demonstrates the neurotransmitter systems that influence these connections, as well as their excitatory or inhibitory influences. Loop I may function to maintain a continuous stream of cognitive and emotional impulses through an essentially positive feedback loop back and forth from the limbic cortex and the dorsomedial nucleus of the thalamus. This loop can be influenced by "outside" inhibition (noradrenergic inhibition from the locus coeruleus, gamma-aminobutyric acid-ergic [GABA-ergic] inhibition from

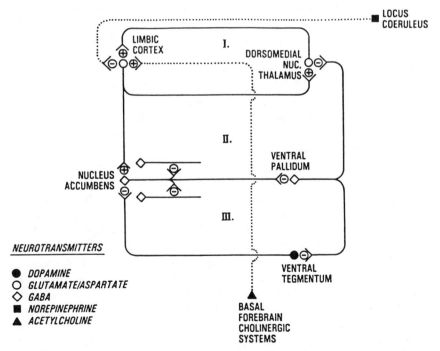

FIGURE 1.4. Normal limbic circuitry in the brain. From Swerdlow & Koob (1987). Copyright 1987 by Cambridge University Press. Reprinted by permission.

the ventroposterior nucleus of the thalamus) or excitation by cholinergic neurotransmission. Loop II operates under the opposing excitatory and inhibitory effects of glutamatergic and GABA-ergic neurons, as well as excitatory effects of one set of inhibitors upon another through disinhibition. Loop III is an entirely negative feedback loop with the inhibitory activity of dopaminergic, glutamatergic, and GABA-ergic neurons.

Through the normal functioning of these circuits, cognitive and emotional information can be modulated in a number of different ways: (1) New patterns can be initiated, (2) irrelevant patterns can be "filtered out," and (3) existing patterns can be "switched." In Swerdlow and Koob's (1987) theoretical model, alterations of this circuitry can result in "pathological" changes relevant to more than one specific disease entity. The disturbance to such circuitry can provide an explanation for depression. A relative lack of DA at the nucleus accumbens (NAC) will disinhibit the inhibitory influence of neurons of the ventroposterior nucleus of the thalamus, leaving loop I in an unchecked positive feedback circuit and leaving the NAC unable to switch or initiate new cognitive sets. Clinically, psychomotor retardation, a paucity of affect, cognitive "rigidity" or perseveration, and anhedonia may be affective analogues of the motor effects from loss of DA activity in those basal ganglionic areas associated with parkinsonism. Indeed, in animal models, depletion of DA from the NAC reduces or eliminates the rewarding effects of sex, food, electrical brain stimulation, and psychostimulants such as cocaine and amphetamine (Swerdlow & Koob, 1987).

Decreased NE activity from the locus coeruleus will disinhibit the corticothalamic activity in a similar fashion, with a reduction in NAC activity. NAC transmission is also associated with activation of the hypothalamic nuclei; these contain CRF, which initiates cortisol activity (see "Cortisol Abnormalities," above). Other hypothalamic functions that are disturbed in depressive states (sleep, appetite, and libido) can be influenced by alterations in this circuitry.

The NAC and temporal lobe structures, including the hippocampus, are major terminal fields for the ascending serotonergic projections from the dorsal and median raphe nuclei. While the behavioral consequences of changes in forebrain 5-HT activity are complex and are less well understood than those of changes in the major DA systems, it is clear that changes in mesolimbic 5-HT transmission have profound effects on corticostriatothalamic function. Some of these effects may result from 5-HT interactions with DA activity within the ventral tegmentum or nucleus accumbens, whereas hippocampal influences of 5-HT may be relatively independent of forebrain DA systems. Indeed, there is substantial preclinical evidence for potent behavioral effects of SSRI-class antidepressants, resulting from their action within both the limbic cortex and the limbic striatum (Swerdlow & Koob, 1987).

Although there is much evidence for the existence and function-ing of this circuitry, the model presented here is speculative as it relates to depressive phenomena. However, it suggests the complexity of the problems faced in unraveling knowledge of this illness.

PSYCHOPHARMACOLOGICAL TREATMENT OF DEPRESSION

The most powerful confirmation of the biological nature of depres-sion has been the dramatic impact of antidepressant pharmacotherapy (Brown & Mann, 1984; Richelson, 1991; Sulser et al., 1978). Psycho-pharmocological studies over the past 40 years have demonstrated the efficacy of antidepressant medications in treating episodes of unipolar major depression, depressive episodes in bipolar disorders, and dysthymic disorders. Although numerous antidepressants are currently available on the market in the United States—drugs that are structurally different, and whose presumed mechanisms of actions are varied—it appears to be the case at present that for a given depressive disorder (with few ex-ceptions), all of the primary antidepressants have equivalent efficacy. Because our purpose is to give the reader a general overview of the psy-chopharmacological treatment of depression, we leave many of the details and subtleties to more comprehensive reviews.

There are four general classes of antidepressant medications, grouped together by both their structural–functional similarities and the history of their development. We review these agents, their dosages (see Table 1.3), and their usual side effects (see Tables 1.4 and 1.5).

Monoamine Oxidase Inhibitors

MAOIs were the first antidepressants to be discovered. There are now two widely used MAOIs: phenelzine (Nardil) and tranylcypromine (Parnate) (Zisook, 1985). Their most common side effects include mild anticholinergic effects, orthostatic hypotension, and sexual dysfunction. At adequate doses, these drugs have been very effective antidepressants. However, they lost favor during the 1960s and 1970s following the reports of numerous hypertensive crises, including some fatal strokes, precipitated by unmetabolized dietary tyramine (an amino acid found in many aged foods, wines, and cheeses). Once the mechanism of this health-threatening reaction was clarified, clinicians were able to caution patients to modify their diets and to avoid sympathomimetic drugs, which also caused such reactions. With proper precautions, these drugs have resumed a role in the armamentarium used to combat depression. Because they are non-specific in their primary effects of inhibiting the oxidation metabolism

TABLE 1.3. Recommended Dosages of Frequently Used Antidepressants

Drug	Usual daily adult dose range (mg)[a]
Tricyclic antidepressants	
Amitriptyline	75–300
Desipramine	75–300
Doxepin	75–300
Imipramine	75–300
Nortriptyline	50–150
Protriptyline	15–60
Trimipramine	50–300
Clomipramine	75–300
Monoamine oxidase inhibitors	
Isocarboxazid	10–50
Phenelzine	45–90
Tranylcypromine	30–60
"Older" second-generation antidepressants	
Amoxapine	150–400
Maprotiline	75–225
Trazodone	150–600
"Newer" second-generation antidepressants	
Bupropion	200–450
Fluoxetine	20–80
Sertraline	50–200
Paroxetine	20–40
Venlafaxine	75–225
Nefazodone	300–600

Note. From Zisook & Andia (1992). Copyright 1992 by Advanstar Communications, Inc. Reprinted by permission.

[a]Usual beginning doses in geriatric patients are one-third to one-half of those used in other adults. Upper range is generally used only for severely depressed, treatment-refractory patients.

of all monoamines, they have a broad spectrum of action, with enhancing effects on the NE, 5-HT, and DA systems (Liebowitz et al., 1988). Presently, several newer, more specific, and reversible MAOIs, with better safety profiles, are being investigated as possible antidepressant agents. One such medication, L-deprenyl, a selective inhibitor of MAO type B, is available for the treatment of Parkinson's disease and may have antidepressant properties. Another, moclobemide, the first of the so-called "reversible inhibitors" of MAO type A, promises to be an effective antidepressant and anxiolytic medication.

TABLE 1.4. Relative Reuptake-Inhibiting Effects and Neurotransmitter Receptor Affinities of Antidepressants

Drug	Reuptake blockade		Receptor affinity[a]			
	NE	5-HT	Ach	H_1	C_1	D_2
	Tricyclic antidepressants					
Amitriptyline	2	2	3	3	4	1
Desipramine	4	0–1	1–2	1	2	1
Doxepin	2	0–1	2	4	4	1
Imipramine	2	2	2	2	3	1
Nortriptyline	3	0–1	2	2	3	1
Protriptyline	4	1	3	2	2	1
Trimipramine	0–1	0	2	4	4	2
Clomipramine	1	3	3	2	3	2
	"Older" second-generation antidepressants					
Amoxapine	3	1	1	2	3	2
Maprotiline	3	0–1	0–1	3	3	1
Trazodone	0–1	2	0	1	4	1
	"Newer" second-generation antidepressants					
Bupropion	0	0	0	0–1	0–1	0
Fluoxetine	1	3	0–1	0–1	0–1	1
Sertraline	1	3	1	0	1	0–1
Paroxetine	1	4	2	0	0–1	0
Venlafaxine	1	2	0	0	0	0
Nefazodone	0–1	1	0	0	3	1

Note. 0 = no affinity; 4 = much affinity. From Richelson & Elliot (1994). Copyright 1994 by *Mayo Clinic Proceedings.* Reprinted by permission.
[a]ACh, acetylcholine; H_1, histamine$_1$; C_1, alpha$_1$; D_2, dopamine$_2$.

Tricyclic Antidepressants

All of the currently available TCAs also have a broad spectrum of action; that is, they have reuptake-blocking effects in both the NE and 5-HT systems (Richelson, 1991), the two neurotransmitter systems most closely linked to depression. Their side effect profiles reflect the fact that they also have substantial affinity for cholinergic, histaminergic, and alpha-adrenergic receptors, accounting for many of their troublesome side effects (see Tables 1.4 and 1.5). Therefore, even with effective treatment patients commonly experience dry mouth, blurred vision, rapid pulse, constipation, urinary retention, sedation, weight gain, and cognitive

TABLE 1.5. Relationship between Pharmacological Properties of Antidepressants and Clinical Actions or Side Effects

Property	Action/side effect
Blockade of NE reuptake	Relief of dysphoria
	Tremors
	Tachycardia
	Disturbances of erection and ejaculation
	Interference with antihypertensive effects of guanethidine and guanadrel
	Augmentation of pressor effects of sympathomimetics
Blockade of muscarinic receptors (cholinergic)	Dry mouth
	Constipation
	Blurred vision
	Tachycardia
	Urinary retention
	Confusion
Blockade of histaminergic receptors	Sedation
	Weight gain
	Hypotension
Blockade of antiadrenergic receptors	Orthostatic hypotension
	Potentiation of antihypertensive effects of antiadrenergic blockers, such as prazosin
	Reflex tachycardia
Blockade of D_2 receptors	Extrapyramidal and endocrinological side effects
	Sexual dysfunction in males
Blockade of 5-HT_2 receptors	Alleviation of rhinitis
	Hypotension
	Migraine headache prophylaxis

Note. From Zisook & Andia (1992). Copyright 1992 by Advanstar Communications, Inc. Reprinted by permission.

disturbances. Until the 1980s, and to a lesser extent today, treatment with antidepressants has involved balancing the beneficial effects in fighting a dreadful disease against the largely "nuisance" problems of side effects (Tollefson, 1991), which can often reach proportions sufficient to limit the treatment. A final and very serious consideration in the use of TCAs is that they are often lethal in overdose.

"Older" Second-Generation Antidepressants

In the early 1980s, three new compounds became available. The first, amoxapine, is a TCA that is a metabolite of the antipsychotic drug loxapine. As a strong NE reuptake blocker, it has the advantages and disadvantages of its parent compound. Its antidopaminergic activity suggests benefits for use with psychotic depression, but also accounts for some of its problematic side effects, including extrapyramidal movement disorders (e.g., tardive dyskinesia) and galactorrhea, in addition to the usual side effects of TCAs (Richelson, 1991; Yassa et al., 1987).

The second antidepressant in this group is maprotiline, an effective and powerful fairly selective tetracyclic noradrenergic agent with milder anticholinergic activity, which makes it well tolerated. However, its popularity has suffered from reports of seizure activity (Dessain et al., 1986), and, like the TCAs, it is lethal in overdose.

Trazodone, another tetracyclic compound, was the first fairly 5-HT-specific antidepressant introduced in the United States. Compared to the TCAs, it has fewer anticholinergic and antihistaminic side effects and has not been fatal in overdose (Tollefson, 1991; Richelson, 1991). However, it has had its own problems, often requiring rather high doses for its antidepressant effects. Because it has potent alpha-adrenergic-blocking activity, it can cause orthostatic hypotension. It is very sedating, and in men may lead to prolonged, painful, and dangerous erection (Tollefson, 1991; Richelson, 1991). A medication that works similarly to trazodone, nefazodone, has recently become available. Nefazodone appears to have the advantages of trazadone without the propensity to disrupt sleep patterns, lead to orthostatic hypotension, or cause priapism (Taylor et al., 1987).

"Newer" Second-Generation Antidepressants

The newest group of antidepressants includes the three SSRIs, fluoxetine, sertraline, and paroxetine, as well as two unique compounds, bupropion and venlafaxine. What characterizes this newest generation of agents is the specificity of many of their actions and, as a corollary, the relative absence of anticholinergic, antihistaminergic, and anti-alpha-adrenergic side effects. This latter property has made these drugs "cleaner" to use, allowing clinicians to target "purer" antidepressant action. These compounds are equivalent in efficacy to one another, as well as to the older drugs. Of great importance to clinicians treating depression is that these new medications present a very limited risk of lethal overdose (Zisook, 1992).

The SSRIs, led by fluoxetine (Prozac), have captured a large percentage of the market, as physicians have preferred to use medicines that are well tolerated (Markowitz, 1991). The most frequent side effects are headaches, nausea, nervousness, insomnia, tremor, and sexual dysfunctions. The three available SSRIs differ somewhat from one another in their particular side effect profiles, active metabolites, and half-lives. For example, fluoxetine has a very long half-life (3–5 days) and a long-acting active metabolite. Paroxetine may be more sedating and less likely to exacerbate nervousness. Physicians often utilize these differences in their selections.

Bupropion, a monocyclic aminoketone, is structurally quite different from other antidepressants (Gardner, 1991). It is also unique in its activity: It neither blocks reuptake of monoamines nor acts on the 5-HT system. It has some noradrenergic activity, as it has been found to decrease noradrenergic firing at the locus coeruleus and to decrease NE turnover. It also has mild dopaminergic activity, which is unlikely to account for its effectiveness as an antidepressant. Its side effects are similar to those of SSRIs and much better tolerated than those of TCAs. Shortly before its release, bupropion was withdrawn when a high incidence of seizures was found in a small group of nondepressed bulimic patients (Sheehan et al., 1986). Subsequent studies showed that the incidence of seizure activity was equivalent to that of other antidepressant medications when the drug was taken in divided doses up to the recommended limit of 450 mg/day (Davidson, 1989).

At this writing, the newest available antidepressant medication is venlafaxine (Montgomery, 1993). It also has a novel structure; its side effect profile is similar to that of the SSRIs, except for some greater sedation and its dose-related association with sustained increases in blood pressure, which requires closer monitoring for the occurrence of hypertension. Its mechanism of action as an antidepressant is also different: In a move back toward a "broader-spectrum" drug, it has properties of both potent 5-HT and NE reuptake inhibition and mild DA inhibition, together with an absence of effects on cholinergic, histaminergic, and alpha-adrenergic receptors. Of all available antidepressant medications, venlafaxine exerts the most rapid downregulation of postsynaptic beta-adrenergic receptors. Whether this translates into a more rapid onset of action than that of other medications has not been demonstrated.

Other Drugs with Antidepressant Properties

Up to this point, we have been describing the properties of medications whose primary uses are for the treatment of depression. However, numerous other drugs have shown some antidepressant activity or have been used in conjunction with antidepressants to enhance their effects. Table 1.6 lists these drugs, together with their primary usages and their roles in treating depression.

TABLE 1.6. Adjunctive Drugs in Treating Depression

Drug	Class	Role in depression
Alprazolam	Anxiolytic	Benefit in low doses in mild depression with anxiety
Buspirone	Anxiolytic	Partial 5-HT agonist with some primary antidepressant effects at high doses (40–60 mg/day) and augmentation of SSRIs, TCAs at moderate doses (30 mg/day)
Selegiline	Antiparkinsonian	Inhibitor of MAO type B in low doses
Lithium	Mood stabilizer	Mild primary effects; adjunctive, augmenting with TCAs, SSRIs
Thyroid hormone	Hormone	Augmentation of other antidepressants
Estrogen	Hormone (antimenopausal)	Augmentation of antidepressants in menopausal women
Methylphenidate/ amphetamine	Stimulant	Adjunctive with TCAs

Electroconvulsive Therapy

Once a mainstay of treatment for severe depression, ECT has been relegated to the status of an emergency procedure for the most seriously suicidal patients or a "last-ditch" effort for refractorily depressed patients in most parts of the United States. This is unfortunate, though quite understandable. From a scientific standpoint, ECT is clearly the most effective treatment for severe major depression (American Psychiatric Association, 1978), with improvement rates approaching 90% (vs. 70% for antidepressant medications). Its disuse has been a product of both its early misuse (it was used in treating every serious form of mental illness) and because of its "primitive" technology, which created a stereotype of "barbarism" associated with it.

Seizure-inducing techniques (insulin administration to cause insulin shock, pentylenetetrazol injection to induce chemical seizures, and ECT) have been used for over 50 years. Until the 1970s, patients undergoing ECT were at risk for sequelae such as pain, fractures, and myocardial infarction, as well as confusion and memory loss. With evolving technology, modern ECT employs unilateral leads, preanesthesia, full general anesthesia, and cardiac and electroencephalographic (EEG) monitoring, so that the patient experiences no physical discomfort and usually only short-term confusion and memory loss. However, residual images of ECT's "barbarism," and mass media portrayals of its use as punishment (as in the novel and film *One Flew Over the Cuckoo's Nest*), have operated to make clinicians reluctant to recommend ECT and patients reluctant to accept it (American Psychiatric Association, 1978).

Summary

There exists a large armamentarium of antidepressant medications whose efficacy is established and unequivocal. Moreover, several drugs used to treat other conditions have antidepressant properties, and ECT is an extremely effective form of treatment. The artful application of scientific knowledge about these powerful agents can improve the lives of as many as 90% of those who suffer from various forms of depression. There are very few chronic illnesses in all of medicine for which such a relatively good prognosis is available.

CONCLUSION: MOVING TOWARD A SYNTHESIS

For many years, science has used the "one gene, one enzyme" approach to guide its research endeavors. In a sense, researchers have been looking for the one "weak link" or "flaw" that causes an illness such as depression. However, with some notable exceptions (e.g., sickle cell anemia), this "weak link" approach to understanding the etiology of clearly multifactorial illnesses such as cardiovascular disease and depressive disorders is too simplistic.

The brain is a biological organ that coordinates a wide range of complex activities. This complexity requires an organ that has built-in plasticity and resilience. Each of the hypotheses described in this chapter describes a way to understand certain pieces of what we know about depression. None of these hypotheses is sufficient to explain fully the complexity and the nuances of depression that clinicians see in their patients on a daily basis. The biological foundations of depression are being approached through a series of successive approximations, moving toward a synthesis from multiple directions. None has hit the mark in an unequivocal fashion, but all are contributing to a broader understanding of what depression seems to be: an autonomous disorder, affected by and affecting numerous systems in the brain and their connections both within the brain and elsewhere in the body.

·2·

Changing Models of Psychopathology

When the plasterboard begins falling from the ceiling, one remedy may be only to replace the plasterboard, which may be somehow inherently defective. Another approach may be to place a drain in the space above the plasterboard and siphon out water, which may be accumulating above and causing pressure upon the ceiling. A third approach may be to repair the leaking roof. The specific remedy applied to this situation depends on one's assessment of the nature of the problem. Before one begins to fix the problem, it is important to know what is wrong.

Throughout the history and traditions of medicine, as well as of antecedent and concurrent practices in other forms of healing arts and in religious and spiritual customs, the central question that precedes any form of intervention is "What's wrong?" Because there are many ways to examine a problem, there are always numerous ways of understanding what is wrong. In medicine, diagnoses have become increasingly refined in their appreciation of underlying pathology. In psychiatry, the past three decades have revolutionized the conceptualization of many forms of psychopathology. This chapter examines the critical conceptual shifts that have occurred as biological models of depression have emerged and begun to coexist with or to supplant earlier psychodynamic models.

PSYCHODYNAMIC MODELS

Prior to the biological revolution, the prevailing school of thought about the nature of psychopathology was psychoanalytic theory as developed by Freud in the 1890s, and modified by him and many others during the first six decades of the 20th century. Psychodynamic models of psychopathology have evolved in a number of directions: orthodox analytic psychology, ego psychology, object relations theory, and self psychology, among others. Each of these psychodynamic models contains an organized, internally consistent, and integrated view of personality development and symptom formation. Although none of these views have demonstrated any external validity that is acceptable to the scientific community, their adherents maintain strong convictions about the wisdom and validity of their belief systems—convictions based on the cleverness and plausibility of the models, the success of their teachers, and the consistency of these models with their own personal and clinical experiences. As a result, psychodynamic theory continues to have a significant influence in the training of psychotherapists and the practice of psychotherapy.

There has been a general trend within training programs to avoid dichotomizing the biological and psychodynamic perspectives or polarizing their adherents. No one wants to "throw out the baby with the bath water," alienate important contributors to teaching and supervision, or appear closed-minded. As a result, we have observed that "integrated" and "eclectic" programs have tended to let adherents of different viewpoints "do their thing" and compete in the marketplace of ideas for the hearts and minds of developing professionals. However, the psychodynamic models contain numerous underlying assumptions about the nature of symptomatic psychopathology that are inconsistent with, and at times diametrically opposed to, the parallel assumptions of a biological framework. We first examine these assumptions from a psychodynamic perspective, and then examine the same tenets and their modification from a biological perspective. Although the focus of this book is on the biology of symptomatic disorders, it should be noted that there is a parallel and increasing research literature on the biology of personality development and disorders.

The basic assumptions of psychodynamic models of psychopathology in symptomatic disorders are as follows:

1. Symptoms are produced by conflict, which is often unconscious.
2. Symptoms have symbolic meaning.
3. Symptoms are equivalent to one another: "Symptoms are symptoms are symptoms."
4. Symptoms are multipotential in nature (i.e., they may be interpreted in many different ways, depending on their context).
5. Character strength is the main factor in prevention of and protection from symptomatic disorders.

The Conflict-Bound Nature of Symptoms

One of the fundamental assumptions of psychodynamic theory is that symptoms are *caused by* conflict, and that often this conflict is unconscious. The "neuroses" (the usual term for most symptoms of anxiety and/ or depression) are seen as manifestations of developmentally higher-level forms of conflict—expressions of "genital" or "Oedipal" conflicts in a psychosexual developmental scheme (Freud, 1905/1953; Brenner, 1955; Fenichel, 1945). Psychotic disorders are considered manifestations of conflict or arrest at the earliest preverbal phases of development, whereas obsessive–compulsive disorders evolve from disruption at the "anal" phase of psychosexual development. Although moderate psychodynamic thinkers have minimized the correlations between symptom formation and stages of psychosexual development, there remains a conviction that symptoms are superficial manifestations of an underlying problem of a psychological nature.

Some of the early formulations of the psychodynamics of depression ascribed its occurrence to unconscious hostility, which keeps the person from being able to love and leads to feelings of guilt, inadequacy, emptiness, and self-hatred (Abraham, 1911/1948). Freud (1917/1957) agreed with Abraham's proposition that depression stems from hostility toward a loved one who has been lost, but added that the loved object is incorporated into the self and that the hostility is then turned toward that part of the self. Depression is thus the result of pathological ambivalence toward a lost love object.

Rado (1927) proposed a variation of this theory, based on the provocative role of the critical superego. The ego reacts to loss with primitive rage and is criticized for this rage, leading to guilt and fear that such rage will destroy the loved object. The ego then punishes itself to prevent the loss of its own superego as well as the lost object. The superego's criticism leads to a sense of worthlessness and guilt, while self-punitive efforts lead to anhedonia, anorexia, and suicide.

Fenichel (1945) extended these theories of depression in suggesting that the loss of a loved one contributes to the lowering of the self-esteem obtained from that relationship. He also said that depression can result from any circumstances that affect self-esteem. Bibring (1953) took this notion a step further, saying that any experience resulting in the ego's perception that it cannot live up to its "ego ideal" will also result in depression.

Each of these psychodynamic models addresses a conflict-bound theme whose essence is causative. A corollary to this theme is that the relationship between symptom and conflict is not only causal, but fluid and continuous. By this we mean that the symptom's presence, level of intensity, and ebb and flow reflect the current status of the conflict. Although conflict may occur without symptom formation, symptoms are always manifestations of conflict. Symptoms are not independent of or dissociated from conflicts.

The Symbolic Nature of Symptoms

The second psychodynamic assumption about symptoms posits a direct connection between the nature of the conflict and the specific manifestation of the symptoms. This view was propounded and supported most vigorously by Freud's work with Breuer in using hypnosis to cure hysterical conversion symptoms (Breuer & Freud, 1893–1895/1955). It was substantiated solely through individual case studies replete with examples of hysterical paralyses, aphonias, and amnesias whose purposes were to protect the patients from awareness of their aggressive and sexual conflicts with significant others (Breuer & Freud, 1893–1895/1955; Janet, 1907/1965; Ludwig, 1971). Once there is an assumption that symptoms behave in this way, it is a simple extension of logic and reasoning to create a level of "understanding" of the meanings and purposes of a symptom, whether the symptom is one of anxiety, depression, or even psychosis.

Another product of this theme is the concept of "secondary gain" (Greenson, 1967; Brenner, 1955). Secondary gain extends the "purpose" of a symptom beyond its primary function of conflict deflection, displacement, or avoidance, and creates an opportunity for the patient to fulfill dependency needs, obtain emotional or financial support, regress, or avoid distressing circumstances. Secondary gain is seen as advantageous to the patient and increases the patient's motivation to maintain symptoms. In most clinical teaching settings we have observed, issues of secondary gain have become a standard element of discussion, at times achieving paramount status.

Symptom Equivalency

In a psychodynamic framework, symptoms as manifestations of underlying conflict may be quite variable in terms of their frequency, intensity, tenacity, chronicity, or relationship in time to their presumed precipitants (Greenson, 1967; Brenner, 1955). On the one hand, the underlying and unresolved conflict that results in symptom formation may be quite dissociated from the symptoms in time, but because the unconscious is "timeless" (Brenner, 1955), the fact of such a conflict's existence is sufficient to explain symptomatic phenomena whenever they may occur. On the other hand, because the unconscious is by definition unknown, the relationship of conflict to all of those qualities that can describe a symptom is accounted for, whether such qualities remain fixed or undergo any number of changes. We can see that a tautology exists— circular thinking, which is its own validation. Thus, anxiety or depression can be short-lived and transient, or persistent, pervasive, and all-consuming, without altering the understanding of its underlying cause. There becomes no need to differentiate the features of a symptom: A symptom is a symptom is a symptom.

The Multipotential Nature of Symptoms

Although psychodynamic theory depicts certain symptom clusters or syndromes as being associated with different levels of psychosexual development, there remains broad latitude in the manner in which phenomenologically similar symptoms may be interpreted, depending on the clinician's perception of the level of the patient's developmental maturation. Symptoms of anxiety may be viewed as features of disintegration in a prepsychotically organized patient. They may also be seen as manifestations of separation anxiety in a person with borderline personality organization; of an acutely threatening and disruptive state in a narcissistically disturbed person's selfobject representation; of anxiety generated by sexual conflicts within a marriage; or of fears about expressing one's rage. Similarly, depressive symptoms may be seen as representing lowered self-esteem following disappointment; the impact of loss of a relationship; anger turned inward; or an anaclitic depression whose roots are in developmental disruption.

In all of these cases, it is the context that defines the essence of each "type" of anxiety or depressive symptom, rather than inherent features of a symptom itself. The essential psychopathology is still defined by parameters that are relatively independent of these symptoms. Furthermore, the views of pathology given above would not be appreciably different if symptoms were switched from one set of conflicts to the other. The anxiety symptoms may be equally applicable to all of the situations with which the depressive symptoms can be linked, and vice versa. Again, the symptomatic picture is almost incidental to what's "really wrong."

The Protective and Preventive Functions of Character

In psychodynamic theory, symptoms represent a breakdown in the defensive functions of character and ego mechanisms (Brenner 1955; Nemiah, 1973). Figure 2.1 schematically depicts the mechanisms by which psychological homeostasis is maintained.

Under ordinary circumstances, psychological conflicts lead to preconscious or signal anxiety, which is managed through the use of automatic and usually unconscious mechanisms of defense. These defenses are hierarchical in nature, reflecting varying degrees of developmental maturation. The first lines of defense are the "most mature" operations, such as the use of humor, altruism, suppression, and sublimation. Should these defen-

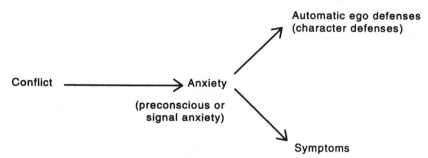

FIGURE 2.1. Mechanisms for maintenance of psychological homeostasis.

sive (and inherently adaptive) mechanisms be ineffective in modifying the conflict-driven anxiety, the "normal" or "neurotic" defenses (e.g., repression, rationalization, displacement, and reaction formation) are initiated. Finally, the more "primitive" and "immature" defenses are enlisted to contain the conflict (e.g., projection, distortion, splitting, and somatization). When all of these resources are ineffective or inadequate, there is a breakthrough of symptoms. This extends the psychodynamic concept of psychopathology of symptom formation to include not just the central role of unresolved conflict, but also a defect in the homeostatic mechanisms represented by the character's defensive structure. "Character weakness," thus defined, becomes a part of the clinical picture of symptomatology. Conversely, the person with a "healthy ego" is relatively invulnerable to developing a psychiatric disorder, and if this is strong enough, it will prevent the development of symptoms.

Contributing to this view is a lack of differentiation between transitory effects of anxiety or depression, which arise specifically out of conflict and do resolve under the mollifying effects of one or other adaptive/defensive operation, and the symptoms that are part of a larger syndrome or disorder. It is also complicated by the reality that one can almost always see connections, either casual or associational, between such symptoms and the psychological matrix in which they are embedded, furthering the view that ego deficits contribute to symptom formation or their perpetuation.

Nemiah (1973) describes the vulnerability of certain personalities to depression:

> It is an illness which afflicts a more limited number of people made susceptible to it by their narcissistic character structure and the ambivalent nature of the human relationships they establish. In them, as in their more normal fellows, lowered self-esteem and loss produce a feeling of

depression, but because of their narcissism and their strong dependent needs, the feeling of depression they suffer is particularly painful. They are especially sensitive to loss which so lowers their self-esteem and increases their psychic pain that it may become intolerable. Because of their abnormal sensitivity, the stimulus that produces such an affect in a narcissistic person may be relatively slight; a mild rebuff or the minor defection of a person they rely on, which in more normal people would cause little or no disturbance, may precipitate as severe a feeling of depression as the loss by death of someone important to them. The pain is further heightened to an unbearable intensity by the anger that stems from their ambivalence. To protect themselves from this pain, they employ abnormal mechanisms of defense (the heritage of early and immature phases of development); denial of the loss leads to a blocking of the process of grief; identification (and its companion, incorporation) leads to an internalization of at least a part of the image of the lost object, resulting in a variety of somatic complaints, violent self-castigation, and suicide. In most patients, the defensive operations are not entirely effective, and one finds a mixture of the painful affect resulting from loss and the effects of the partly successful defense mechanisms. In other words, in the predisposed individual, the *affect* of depression, which is a normal response to loss and lowered self-esteem, is complicated by additional psychological factors which conspire to produce the *illness*, depression. (pp. 195–196; emphasis in original)

BIOLOGICAL MODELS

It is essential to preface any discussion of the current understanding of biological processes in psychopathology with the recognition that the hypotheses for which some validity has been established through scientific study are tentative, despite the numerous lines of evidence that may seem to substantiate them (see Chapter 1). With that warning, we proceed to examine such models as if they are valid, and then compare and contrast elements of these models with corresponding elements of psychodynamic models.

The concepts central to biological models of psychopathology in symptomatic disorders are as follows:

1. Psychiatric illness represents brain disorder.
2. Symptoms have variable origins and significance.
3. Symptomatic disorders have a variable relationship to life stresses.
4. The interactions of personality and developmental issues with symptomatic disorders are complex.

Psychiatric Illness as Brain Disorder

Despite its oversimplification, the concept of psychiatric illness as brain disorder represents the essence of biological psychiatry and parallels many aspects of the concepts of disease in medicine as a whole. As discussed in Chapter 1, most of the major psychiatric disorders, including depressive disorders, demonstrate genetic vulnerability. This is usually assumed to be a gene-based abnormality of biochemical functioning, with variable penetrability and manifest (phenotypic) expression. Although the "underlying cause" of such a disorder may lie in a biochemical error, the symptoms are seen as constituting the primary clinical disorder. There is no assumption that specific psychological problems "cause" the disorder, though they may contribute as stressors, along with temperamental and other factors, provoking the clinical manifestations of the disorder as a final common pathway (Akiskal & McKinney, 1975; Kendler et al., 1993).

As in many other medical diseases, the behavioral "end-organ" manifestations may be the only or predominant phenomena available for direct observation and examination. Although some brain metabolites are accessible in body fluids (urine, blood, cerebrospinal fluid), and some aspects of brain structure and function can be examined (via MRI, CT, EEG, PET, SPECT), *in vivo* examination (via brain biopsy) is rare and limited to more purely neurobiological and life-threatening disorders. Most psychiatric diagnoses are based on patients' and others' reports and on clinicians' observations of signs and symptoms.

Within a biological model, a syndromatic group of symptoms *is* the disorder with which a patient and clinician must contend. The psychopathology is defined by the symptom manifestations and their impact on the person. Every disorder has a range of characteristics—a set of symptoms, a natural history, an inherited predisposition, and a vulnerability to stressors—that seems to operate within each individual in partly stereotypic and partly idiosyncratic fashion, but is always interwoven with the fabric of preexisting personality development, and at times plays a critical role in that development.

Variable Origins and Significance of Symptoms

Although the number of people who have a diagnosable symptomatic disorder (e.g., major depression or panic disorder) may be limited, some symptoms of anxiety and depression are fairly universal and may represent a number of pathways utilizing both "biological" and "psychological" mechanisms.

Symptoms Arising from Biologically "Wired" Reflexes

In the face of a reality-based immediate threat, manifestations of anxiety as a reaction to imminent danger are highly adaptive as a preparation for fight or flight (Selye, 1950). They serve self- and species-preservative functions and require little more than the perception of danger for their activation. Similarly, features of depression are characteristic and species-specific in response to losses of or separation from significant others (Bowlby, 1973). Neither of these types of responses requires higher levels of perception, symbolic interpretation, or other attribution for their activation, although both types of mechanisms invariably become secondarily complicated by such processes once they have occurred. People will probably attribute whatever meaning they can to such events in order to reestablish homeostasis. For example, although the species-specific response to a loss may involve some social withdrawal, emotional constriction, feelings of sadness, or tearfulness, most people will wonder why the loss occurred, may become angry about it, may feel personally responsible for their suffering, or may begin to rationalize away their pain. It is clear that few primitive paleocortical or mesolimbic systems will operate without activation of neocortical responses. It is likely that the reverse is also true.

Symptoms Arising from Psychological Trauma

An effort is made here to distinguish between some of the manifestations of anxiety or depression that arise from an individual's interpretation of events and those stemming from more instinctive responses. Once the interpretation is made and meaning is attributed to the specific circumstances, more reflexive responses—whether anxious or depressed ones—are likely to occur. Criticism by one's boss may lead to anxiety that the boss could become violent, or may be focused on the possible loss of one's job and the question of one's ability to survive. It may also lead to depressive symptoms based on loss of self-esteem, suppressed anger, or the perception of the ending of that relationship. In such instances, the mechanisms for such responses are built into the person's "wiring," but require specific attribution of meaning to be triggered.

Symptoms Arising from Perturbations of Psychological Processes

Both of the mechanisms described above seem to reflect "normal" processes in which symptoms of anxiety or depression may emerge. There are also people who seem to be psychologically predisposed either to triggering symptomatic responses by misinterpreting perceptions and over-estimating their significance, or to having a habitual response pattern of overreactivity in the face of threats or insults (i.e., reactivity at a much lower threshold than for other people).

Examples of the former pattern, a type of hypersensitivity, can be seen in those people whose early relationships have distorted their capacity to see acceptance, nurturance, or admiration in others, but have fostered views of rejection, exploitation, and self-deprecation, leading to frequent experiences of transient forms of anxiety or depressive symptoms. This susceptibility to injury further undermines these people's self-confidence and creates a sense of insecurity about any approach to new relationships and experiences. Such people are generally seen as personality-disordered or self-disordered. Their experiences may lead to the perpetuation of notions that personality characteristics may predispose these persons to symptomatic disorders. We think it is critical to underscore that these forms of vulnerability result in emotional upset, *not* clinical depression; that is, these are transient states of symptomatic distress that are modifiable through the usual adaptive mechanisms (or, as we shall discuss later, through psychotherapeutic interventions).

Examples of the pattern of overreactivity described above can be seen in those people who have seemingly exaggerated or catastrophic responses to minor insults. The "pump has been primed" by prior experiences, to the degree that such persons' responses appear to be habitual. The psychological notion of "learned helplessness" (Seligman, 1975) reflects these individuals' inclination to move readily into a position of passivity, despair, and inadequacy—an inclination that may have been fostered by early life experiences. Similarly, the biological concept of "kindling" may represent a parallel neurophysiological mechanism. Stressors may trigger the firing of associative pathways that recreate altered states of mind, which perhaps include "flashbacks" of altered perceptions of a psychotic nature, depressive states, or other regressive phenomena. As biological research into psychopathology progresses, the psychological and neurophysiological elements of such states may well come to be seen as simply different measures of the same phenomena. Finally, like hypersensitive responses, hyperreactive responses also tend to be relatively short-lived and changeable, and should not be mistaken for more constant and autonomous disordered states.

Symptoms as Manifestations of an Autonomous Disorder

An essential feature of any biological disorder in medicine is that a primary end organ is malfunctioning, and that this malfunction usually leads to other systemic pathological responses. Most of the time, we are able to see and comprehend only the surface phenomena of a disorder. Thus, in multiple sclerosis, the end organ being affected is the myelin sheath around structures of the central nervous system, and the manifestations of the disease are the myriad neurological and psychiatric symptoms that can occur. Although numerous factors (e.g., genetics, autoimmunity, slow viruses) have been postulated as causative, the demyelinization defines the disorder's clinical appearance. Similarly, atherosclerotic coronary vascular disease may have many contributing factors (e.g., genetics, fat consumption, stress), but the end-organ change—the blockage of coronary vessels—then exerts its influence on the heart's function in ways that become independent of the factors that may have produced the disease. Whether one examines cancer, arthritis, ulcers, or the common cold, there is a point in time at which contributing factors are transformed into the disease process, which then exhibits a life of its own.

Psychiatric disorders have been and remain among the more difficult medical disorders to comprehend. In Chapter 1, we have examined many of the technological advances that have "opened up" previous obstacles to knowledge. Many factors have complicated the understanding of the end organ—the brain. The first of these is that the brain is the organ that is studying itself. It is the most prized human possession, and, because of this, the source of the greatest degree of vulnerability if a person feels it may be disordered. The unacceptability of this personal vulnerability has played an enormous role in the stigmatization of the mentally ill within societies throughout the ages. It has also played a role in the development of theories that have posited control of the disorders within the sufferers themselves—an enormously appealing and reassuring notion. This mechanism, a function of human narcissism and the need for omnipotence and control, continues to play an important role in the resistance that hinders the spread of scientific knowledge. However, people cannot control the processes that make them ill simply by effort or force of will; nor does the sun revolve around the earth.

Aside from technological and psychological factors, the study of the brain and its functions in psychiatric disorders is hampered by the fact that people tend to be increasingly educated and psychologically minded in observing themselves and others. Even where a disorder has acquired a life of its own, it is difficult to distinguish the manifestations of the disorder from the often complex matrix of long-standing intrapsychic conflicts, recent and current life stressors, and adaptive responses to such a disorder. This is especially true because the same kinds of phenomena—emotional states, perceptual and cognitive patterns, and behaviors—form the "language" for translating all of these various elements.

What we are left with in order to define a disordered state as autonomous are not simply the symptoms of the disorder, but their stereotypy, their persistence and consistency over time, and often their refractoriness to the usual efforts which can modify transient symptoms. At present, the DSM-IV (see Chapter 3) has become the "bible" for diagnosing major psychiatric disorders. However, all experienced clinicians recognize its limitations in distinguishing diagnosable autonomous disorders, in which symptoms present in the context of acute stressors, personality-related vulnerabilities, and adaptive or maladaptive responses. Yet the implications for diagnoses and treatment are far-reaching and depend on clinicians' interpretations of such complex clinical phenomena.

Variable Relationship of Life Stressors to Symptomatic Disorders

During the 20th century, there has been a persistent and largely valid notion that life stressors may precipitate many medical disorders—that there exists a mind–body continuum that can be applied to our understanding of psychiatric disturbances. This view has been supported by research in psychosomatic medicine. Life stressors have been quantified, and studies have demonstrated unequivocally that they can contribute to the development of heart disease, gastroenterological disorders, some cancers, and endocrine disturbances, as well as to schizophrenia, unipolar depression, and anxiety disorders (see, e.g., Stroebe & Stroebe, 1987; Brown & Harris, 1989).

The power of life stressors has been shown to lie in the cumulative, *nonspecific* contributions of both positive and negative experiences of an individual. The impact of such forces in transforming the transient emotionally upsetting states into an autonomous disorder is not understood. It is clear, however, that the disorder (e.g., depression) may persist for an extended period of time beyond the point when the immediate impact of the stressor subsides. These phenomena may become quite dissociated. The fact that the depression persists does not mean that the precipitating events are still active stressors, although they may be. For instance, depression stemming from the ending of a relationship may last far beyond the adjustment to this event. As another example, a depression triggered by the loss of a job may persist despite the person's finding a new one, or may be aggravated by the continuing effects of lasting unemployment (e.g., financial stresses, loss of self-esteem, and excessive free time to worry).

Panic disorder or depression can also occur "out of the blue." Despite the usual findings of stressors as significant factors in the development of a symptomatic disorder, they are not prerequisites. People with strong genetic predispositions are more likely to experience symptomatic disorders in the face of lesser degrees of stress. (No one lives in a stress-free environment.) In such people, the diathesis appears to operate on more internal biological variables. Furthermore, for individuals who have recurrent depressive (and other symptomatic) disorders, repeated episodes appear to require lesser degrees of stress (or sometimes none) for their precipitation (Post et al., 1981).

Symptomatic disorders can also *cause* life stressors. The debilitating effects of anxiety and depression can disrupt one's relationships, interfere with work functioning, and produce major upheavals in every aspect of living. A cycle of disorder and dysfunction that feeds on itself quite destructively can develop. An appreciation of this impact will enable the clinician to sort out some of the complex "chicken-and-egg" puzzles that present themselves in patient's histories.

Complex Interactions of Symptomatic Disorders with Personality and Developmental Issues

In contrast to psychodynamic models of psychopathology, in which symptomatic disorders are viewed largely as products of personality-related conflicts and developmental themes, biological models see the symptomatic disorders themselves as the primary and fundamental problems. In biological models, the greatest "weight" or power in the transformation of "normal" life into illness or disorder has been shifted from those factors associated with intrapsychic conflict, external stress, and developmental arrest or turmoil to the factors of individual genetic vulnerability (Kendler et al., 1992). The former continue to be important factors in understanding psychiatric illness, but they are not as prominent or as highly specific or symbolic as in psychodynamic models.

The complex relationship between symptomatic disorders and developmental and personality factors is evident in four separate though overlapping ways:

1. Personality and developmental issues contribute to the expression of symptomatic disorders, but are not the primary forces in their etiology.
2. Personality and developmental issues shape the manifestations of a symptomatic disorder.
3. Personality and developmental issues determine the adaptive and maladaptive responses of an individual experiencing a symptomatic disorder.
4. Symptomatic disorders exert short-term effects upon personality characteristics, and in cases where the diathesis is chronic or starts early in life, it can produce profound developmental distortions.

Etiology of Disorders

Beliefs about the contributions of personality and development as etiological agents in symptomatic disorders have changed in recent years, as noted above. Personality and development have lost their central role as "causes" of these disorders, even though the conflicts and turmoil emanating from these domains can be productive of elaborate and complex transient symptomatology. At times this symptomatic turmoil occurs with sufficient frequency and regularity that it appears to have a life of its own. Conversely, in case where persistent symptoms of an anxiety or depressive disorder are interacting regularly with personality factors, it can be difficult to discern what came first, and the diagnosis of the disorder may be tentative.

Intrapsychic conflicts may help to precipitate a disorder, or may aggravate or intensify its symptoms. In vulnerable individuals, however, the generic and nonspecific stress generated is what produces or enhances the symptoms, and neither the kind of issue (e.g., Oedipal struggle or counterdependency) nor the symbolic nature of the conflict is important. The lessened importance of these factors is difficult for many traditionalists to accept, both because of their centrality in dynamic theory and because of the intellectual spice and challenge that they have provided. It can be extremely gratifying to establish such mysterious connections, as well as self-validating of the critical skills that have been mastered in this belief system. Many psychodynamically oriented clinicians thus resist biological views, despite the findings of basic research, the efficacy of biological treatment studies, and the absence of studies demonstrating an etiological role of psychodynamics in symptom formation.

Part of the problem is that all of human life proceeds in a psychodynamic context. People are born to dependency and inadequacy, and struggle to achieve autonomy and mastery. Relationships are marked by struggles with control and submission, intimacy, fears of rejection, shame and guilt, hostility, sexual conflict, and so on. No set of circumstances, no point in development, no symptomatic phenomenon can occur outside of such a context. If a clinician's fundamental beliefs are that dynamic issues are primarily productive of autonomous symptoms, the tautology inherent in these beliefs can always prevail. There will always be dynamic forces that "explain" the symptoms.

Regarding the role of personality as a predisposing factor in the development of anxiety or depressive disorders, a number of studies suggest that the biological substrate of anxiety and depressive disorders is manifested quite early in development, in the guise of such personality characteristics as temperament, sociability, and cognitive styles. These studies point toward a view of such symptomatic disorders as being poten-tially present "in the wiring" (Kagan et al., 1988; Akiskal, 1990).

Shaping of a Disorder

Personality and developmental issues are powerful forces shaping the clinical picture seen in depressive and anxiety disorders. Although the core symptoms of these disorders seek expression largely in their "raw" forms (anxiety, anergy, anhedonia, insomnia), many of the symptoms are interwoven with "old" issues and themes (e.g., dependency, inadequacy, and intimacy) in a regressive fashion. Regressive personality character-istics may emerge or become exaggerated under the influence of a disor-der. It is useful to consider the effect of superimposing the manifesta-tions of depression or anxiety upon someone who is already struggling (perhaps even quite successfully) with a personal or developmental issue. Even the healthiest and most adaptive person will experience some dis-tortion of himself or herself in a regressive direction. Persistent symp-toms of anxiety and/or depression will invariably have a negative effect, usually in the direction of those conflicts or themes about which the individual is most vulnerable. In a general state of emotional turmoil, there will be a recruitment of old grief, insecurities, self-deprecation, or despair. The sense of being out of control will trigger old feelings of help-lessness, dependency, and inadequacy. Every individual has an idiosyn-cratic set of developmental conflicts, which will appear in their more regressed forms in the context of an ongoing psychiatric disorder. The disorder is not a product of these conflicts, but is a powerful force in recruiting or driving such phenomena.

Adaptive and Maladaptive Responses to a Disorder

Although there may be no degree of personality strength that can pro-tect an individual from developing a symptomatic disorder, all of a person's adaptive capacities can be mobilized in coping with the impact of such a disorder. Developmental experiences of mastery, counterphobic inclinations, a persistent determination, and "strong enough" self-esteem will help to combat the powerful forces of symptoms and regressive pulls. Individuals may not be able to control their emotional states, but they may be able to contain them, tolerate them, and occasionally override them. The ability to sustain high-level coping mechanisms (e.g., ratio-nalization, sublimation, humor) reflects such strength. However, with intensifying symptoms, even the healthiest and most adaptive may suc-cumb to the power of the disorder. Conversely, those who tend to use less adaptive, less mature means of coping with turmoil are likely to be-

come more regressed, with despair, self-deprecation, and acting out occurring sooner and in response to lesser degrees of depression or anxiety. The overt manifestations of a disorder do *not* reflect the inner resources of the individual in terms of the development of the disorder,
but become quite important in the same person's ability to cope with it.

Effects of Symptomatic Disorders on Personality Characteristics

In the late 1960s, there was a clinical "rule of thumb" in working with
adolescents and young adults, which could be paraphrased as follows:
"If you see depression, think of schizophrenia." This view reflected the
belief that depression was a disorder that began in the late third and early
fourth decades of life. Epidemiological studies now make it clear that both
depressive and anxiety disorders are evident quite early in life and are
increasingly common in children and adolescents (Regier et al., 1993).
As a result, clinicians have begun to scrutinize childhood emotional
disturbances with a much higher index of suspicion for depressive as
well as anxiety disorders. There is not only a continued focus on those
developmental issues, conflicts, and trauma that help to shape the growing child, but also an increasing examination of how personality development is shaped by a concurrent symptomatic disorder.

Depression or anxiety invariably has a short-term, state-dependent,
and frequently regressive influence upon the adult personality (Weissman
et al., 1974). When adults are in the throes of such a chronic disorder,
they may develop significant and sustained distortions of their self-concept,
interpersonal relations, and general functioning, even when they have
previously achieved "mature" status in each of these spheres (Agosti
et al., 1991). When the symptomatic disorder subsides, these state-
dependent features will often revert to their "healthier" status, at times
spontaneously and at times with some psychotherapeutic help (Hirschfeld
et al., 1983, 1989).

The situation is much more extreme in children and adolescents.
Persistent depression and/or anxiety, aside from the inherent suffering
it entails, can interfere substantially with any and every phase of normal
development—hampering, distorting, or arresting every element of evolving self-concept, intellectual and cognitive development, or interpersonal
and intrapsychic development. This is compounded by the relative im-
maturity of children's coping skills, and therefore the greater likelihood
of their being overwhelmed by, succumbing to, and regressing in the face
of their disorder. Under such circumstances, we see one of the more
dramatic "turnabouts" in emphasis in the shift to biological models from

traditional dynamic models—that is, "how illness disturbs development" instead of "how development leads to illness."

Although this issue of developmental disturbance is of greatest impact during early development, the clinician must examine similar, though less profound, effects during adult development. People are particularly vulnerable to developmental distortions when the disorder they experience is of a chronic, unremitting type. In such circumstances, both the acute and chronic effects of anxiety or depression on personality functioning can be enormous and devastating (Hirschfeld et al., 1989; Kovacs et al., 1984, 1994).

·3·

The Symptoms
of Depression

The term "depression" has been employed to describe many forms of human experience. Its use has been so widespread, and it may cover so many forms of subjective distress, that there is usually some advantage to examining the specific meaning of the word in a given situation. First, "depression" is a term in common usage for an acute state of upset—one in which a person may have been disappointed, harassed, or rejected, or may have suffered a loss accompanied by sadness and hurt. This state is considered normal, short-lived, responsive to immediate environmental stimuli, and reversible in the face of other environmental changes.

A second meaning of "depression" is a pervasive and persistent mood that is abnormal and is associated with numerous psychiatric, medical, and toxic disorders. This mood state is variously charac-terized by a number of features, including sadness, emptiness, and anhedonia.

In its third sense, "depression" is an autonomous syndrome, disorder, or illness in which mood symptoms may be prominent or central, but to which many other features contribute as well. Depression as a clinical disorder has come to be diagnosed by means of all these associated features, and although it is actually likely to be a heterogeneous group of disorders, the current state of knowledge limits efforts at classification.

Historically, efforts to classify depression were made through clinical observations that lacked sufficient uniformity for systematic study. This resulted in an expansive list of often overlapping types of depression, including a number of dichotomous classifications: "psychotic" versus "neurotic" depression, "retarded" versus "agitated" depression, "endogenous" versus "reactive" depression, and "unipolar" versus "bipolar" depression.

In addition, there were descriptions of "postpartum," "chronic," "paranoid," "neurasthenic," "masked," "involutional," "seasonal," and "atypical" depressions. Each of these classifications described some unique characteristics, as well as the features common to most depressions (Freedman et al., 1975).

The development of the *Diagnostic and Statistical Manual of Mental Disorders* (DSM) by the American Psychiatric Association has been a continuing effort to clarify the classification of mental disorders in order to aid methodology in research, as well as to make the clinical communications among professionals in general more precise. The evolution of this process, as demonstrated in the most recent edition of the DSM (DSM-IV; American Psychiatric Association, 1994), has contributed greatly to our present understanding of the disorders that we clinicians encounter in our work with patients. The use of the highly specific criteria in DSM-IV should yield a greater degree of refinement in research methods and further clarification of the nature of such different syndromes as major depressions, bipolar disorders, dysthymia, seasonal affective disorders, and depressions associated with premenstrual, postpartum, or menopausal changes in women.

DSM-IV CRITERIA

It is useful to begin with a presentation of the DSM-IV criteria for the two primary depressive conditions—major depressive episode and the milder dysthymic disorder. Table 3.1 gives the criteria for the former, and Table 3.2 lists those for the latter. We should note for clarity that major depressive episode is not a codable diagnosis in and of itself, but serves as a "building block" for diagnoses of major depressive disorder and other mood disorders. Depending on a particular patient's history, major depressive disorder may be diagnosed as either "single episode" or "recurrent," and a variety of specifiers may be applied to describe the present or most recent episode: specifiers indicating severity, presence of psychotic features, and remission status; chronicity; presence of catatonic, melancholic, or atypical features; postpartum onset; longitudinal course; and seasonal pattern.

Individual patients will inevitably differ in their types of symptoms, the symptoms' particular forms of expression or the manner in which they are experienced, and symptom severity and persistence. The clinical tasks of exploring these symptoms and determining their autonomy and validity for diagnostic purposes can become quite complicated, even though the DSM-IV looks at times like a cookbook.

TABLE 3.1. DSM-IV Criteria for Major Depressive Episode

A. Five (or more) of the following symptoms have been present during the same 2-week period and represent a change from previous functioning; at least one of the symptoms is either (1) depressed mood or (2) loss of interest or pleasure.

Note: Do not include symptoms that are clearly due to a general medical condition, or mood-incongruent delusions or hallucinations.

    (1) depressed mood most of the day, nearly every day, as indicated by either subjective report (e.g., feels sad or empty) or observation made by others (e.g., appears tearful). **Note:** In children and adolescents, can be irritable mood.

    (2) markedly diminished interest or pleasure in all, or almost all, activities most of the day, nearly every day (as indicated by either subjective account or observation made by others)

    (3) significant weight loss when not dieting or weight gain (e.g., a change of more than 5% of body weight in a month), or decrease or increase in appetite nearly every day. **Note:** In children, consider failure to make expected weight gains.

    (4) insomnia or hypersomnia nearly every day

    (5) psychomotor agitation or retardation nearly every day (observable by others, not merely subjective feelings of restlessness or being slowed down)

    (6) fatigue or loss of energy nearly every day

    (7) feelings of worthlessness or excessive or inappropriate guilt (which may be delusional) nearly every day (not merely self-reproach or guilt about being sick)

    (8) diminished ability to think or concentrate, or indecisiveness, nearly every day (either by subjective account or as observed by others)

    (9) recurrent thoughts of death (not just fear of dying), recurrent suicidal ideation without a specific plan, or a suicide attempt or a specific plan for committing suicide

B. The symptoms do not meet criteria for a Mixed Episode. . . .

C. The symptoms cause clinically significant distress or impairment in social, occupational, or other important areas of functioning.

D. The symptoms are not due to the direct physiological effects of a substance (e.g., a drug of abuse, a medication) or a general medical condition (e.g., hypothyroidism).

E. The symptoms are not better accounted for by Bereavement, i.e., after the loss of a loved one, the symptoms persist for longer than 2 months or are characterized by marked functional impairment, morbid preoccupation with worthlessness, suicidal ideation, psychotic symptoms, or psychomotor retardation.

TABLE 3.2. DSM-IV Criteria for Dysthymic Disorder

A. Depressed mood for most of the day, for more days than not, as indicated either by subjective account or observation by others, for at least 2 years. **Note:** In children and adolescents, mood can be irritable and duration must be at least 1 year.

B. Presence, while depressed, of two (or more) of the following:

  (1) poor appetite or overeating
  (2) insomnia or hypersomnia
  (3) low energy or fatigue
  (4) low self-esteem
  (5) poor concentration or difficulty making decisions
  (6) feelings of hopelessness

C. During the 2-year period (1 year for children or adolescents) of the disturbance, the person has never been without the symptoms in Criteria A and B for more than 2 months at a time.

D. No Major Depressive Episode . . . has been present during the first 2 years of the disturbance (1 year for children and adolescents); i.e., the disturbance is not better accounted for by chronic Major Depressive Disorder, or Major Depressive Disorder, In Partial Remission.
  Note: There may have been a previous Major Depressive Episode provided there was a full remission (no significant signs or symptoms for 2 months) before development of the Dysthymic Disorder. In addition, after the initial 2 years (1 year in children or adolescents) of Dysthymic Disorder, there may be superimposed episodes of Major Depressive Disorder, in which cases both diagnoses may be given when the criteria are met for a Major Depressive Episode.

E. There has never been a Manic Episode . . . , a Mixed Episode . . . , or a Hypomanic Episode . . . , and criteria have never been met for Cyclothymic Disorder.

F. The disturbance does not occur exclusively during the course of a chronic Psychotic Dsorder, such as Schizophrenia or Delusional Disorder.

G. The symptoms are not due to the direct physiological effects of a substance (e.g., a drug of abuse, a medication) or a general medical condition (e.g., hypothyroidism).

Specify if:
  Early Onset: if onset is before age 21 years
  Late Onset: if onset is age 21 years or older
Specify (for most recent 2 years of Dysthymic Disorder):
  With Atypical Features . . .

Note. Reprinted with permission from the *Diagnostic and Statistical Manual of Mental Disorders*, Fourth Edition. Copyright 1994 American Psychiatric Association.

ASSESSING DEPRESSIVE SYMPTOMS FROM
A BIOLOGICAL PERSPECTIVE

The assessment of the symptoms of depression takes on a particular quality when the clinician adopts a biological perspective. Central to this view is that a fundamental series of physiological and biochemical processes has been changed to produce a *continuous* altered state. Independent of the features that contribute to our understanding of what is "biological" about depression (Chapter 1), this perspective entails seeing many of the core elements as superimposed upon a person who is unique by virtue of genetics, development, aesthetics (needs, desires, and tastes), and environmental circumstances. The effort to sort out some variable quantity of a depressive "entity" from the underlying person becomes quite complex and only allows for approximations of understanding. Our experience has been that a biological perspective does not simplify and reduce the elements that need to be taken into account, but adds to the complexity of clinical understanding. Psychological events are by no means eliminated from consideration; they are contributory to, interactive with, and produced by biological events. What are reduced are (1) the "weight" of psychological factors as a necessary precondition of a depressive illness, and (2) the relevance of significant psychological precipitants once a depressive illness has become autonomous (and thereby dissociated from precipitants). What is expanded is the role of biological factors in understanding the psychological *consequences*, both short- and long-term, of a depressive illness.

As we examine the specific symptoms, aware that they often reflect biological changes in the neuroregulatory centers of the hypothalamus, it is with the assumption that most neuroregulatory mechanisms do not operate as all-or-none phenomena but on a continuum of activity. This means that depressive phenomena demonstrate variability in time and intensity except in the most extreme conditions, and that the purposes of assessment are to determine inclinations (is something wrong?), specific functional disturbance (what's wrong?), and intensity of this disturbance (how wrong?).

To illustrate the variability of depressive symptoms, Table 3.3 depicts the differing lifetime prevalences of such symptoms in the general population, as determined by an NIMH epidemiological study.

MOOD SYMPTOMS

There is no single way for mood symptoms of depression to present themselves. People with depression often experience a relatively mild, perva-

TABLE 3.3. Depressive Symptoms: Lifetime Prevalences

	% reporting symptoms lasting 2 weeks or longer	
Symptom	Men	Women
Dysphoria	24	36
Appetite disturbance	19	29
Sleep disturbance	18	27
Psychomotor disturbance	8	10
Loss of interest	3	7
Fatigue	12	20
Guilt	9	12
Diminished concentration	11	17
Thoughts of death	23	33

Note. Data from Robins & Regier (1991).

sive sense of sadness, in the form of feeling low or blue. At the other extreme, there may be an exquisitely painful sense of anguish, which is experienced as all-consuming and never-ending. Or a depressed person may feel empty, emotionally impoverished, or even detached and shut off from feelings; the last of these states is a probable compensatory and self-preservative adaptation to more primary affects. Finally, the dominant mood, especially in a child or adolescent, may be one of irritability, which expresses itself primarily in interactions with others. At times, this irritability may present itself in the earliest phases of a major depressive episode and serve as a signal to the person or those around him or her that depression has returned.

For most people, there is an awareness of a change in mood, but this is not universal. Typically, people will say that they feel different or "I'm not myself." It is not unusual for a mood state to change and "carry" a person with it; the mood change exerts its effects, but without the individual's registering the change. This loss of the observing ego may not reflect an individual's usual capacity at all. On the contrary, the depressive state is likely to be responsible for the person's "capture." This notion of being a "captive" of an altered state is an important point to which we will return many times. Another variant of this process occurs when an individual recognizes elements of depressed or irritable mood but attributes them to immediate environmental stimuli, rendering them irrelevant to the person. The mood is presented as related to existential issues, self-evident, almost ego-syntonic: "Anyone would feel this way under the circumstances." As a result, such an individual may be less likely to endorse the presence of a mood change, but remain focused on the circumstances: "The world is a depressing place, though I am not depressed."

The tasks for the clinician trying to identify and clarify mood symptoms can range in difficulty from "child's play" to the heights of exasperation. Some patients who are highly educated about depression will present with a self-defined, clearly described picture of a mood change "out of the blue" or "like a cloud passed over me," which has been persistent and distressing. Despite the apparent clarity and insight of such observations, some clinicians (i.e., clinicians without a biological perspective) will interpret such presentations as the patients' efforts to deal with depression as an entity unrelated to themselves or to avoid dealing with the "real issues."

Conversely, when a patient presents with a picture of existential depression, it is quite common for the clinician to get caught up in the "existentiality" without considering whether the mood change may still be part of a depression. Although many issues are upsetting, *no human experience is inherently "depressing"* in the sense that it invariably causes clinical depression. More than half of those who have lost a spouse do *not* become depressed, for example. Thus, the clinician must still determine whether a mood symptom has achieved autonomy.

This determination is further complicated by the fact that depressive symptoms may persist over time without actually achieving autonomy. The DSM-IV (American Psychiatric Association, 1994) has defined this situation as an "adjustment disorder with depressed mood." A person may exhibit depressive symptoms for a period of up to 3 months following a specific psychosocial stressor without qualifying for a diagnosis of major depressive disorder. Since many events can be understood as stressors sufficient to precipitate such symptoms, there is still the opportunity to attribute symptoms to an adjustment disorder rather than to major depression. Furthermore, many stressors are persistent and can continue to aggravate or exacerbate such symptoms (e.g., severe financial distress, homelessness).

Yet another factor that complicates the assessment of mood is that except in the most severe depressive states, where mood is considered "unreactive" or refractory to any immediate interventions (personal contact, empathy, etc.), most depressed people can either identify some circumstances in which their mood is responsive and changeable, or demonstrate some mood reactivity in the interview in response to interactions with or qualities of the clinician.

Finally, patients may be reluctant to share the depth of their mood with another person, including the clinician to whom they have gone (or been sent) for help. They may feel too vulnerable, ashamed, or humiliated to express these feelings. This may be accompanied by a very capable performance of "hiding" their feelings from the clinician as they have done in the rest of life, by "putting on a happy face" or generating the appearance of a better mood. Other cases in which people may not accurately communicate their mood are as follows: (1) Adolescents tend to be less expressive and more likely to act upon their feelings; (2) the very old may present with more cognitive dysfunction or somatic symptoms and have a limited focus on unhappiness or sadness; and (3) for the medically ill, somatic symptoms often overshadow affective ones.

All of these factors can complicate the assessment of mood symptoms as part of a clinical depression. It is usually relatively easy to determine their existence, but much more difficult and at times impossible to determine whether the mood disturbance has become autonomous. Fortunately, there are several other clinical variables to assess.

VEGETATIVE SYMPTOMS

Traditionally, such vegetative symptoms as sleep and appetite disturbances, diminished energy, and fatigue have been seen as indications of the severity of a depressive episode. Increasingly, there is evidence that these symptoms may make their appearance quite early in the evolution of a depressive episode; this is particularly true of sleep disturbances.

Sleep Disturbances

Sleep disturbances take various forms (Gillin et al., 1984). People with depression often have diminished sleep. They may have problems with falling asleep, often ruminating about their troubles. Sleep architecture changes in depression include a shortened REM latency, increased REM sleep, and diminished deep sleep (stages 3 and 4). Depressed patients are also likely to have frequent awakenings, and often awaken 2–3 hours before their usual morning awakening time without being able to return to sleep. Aside from any other primary elements of depression, the fatigue and inefficiency secondary to lack of sleep may become important factors in assessment.

A common variant of sleep disturbance is hypersomnia. Some patients describe the inclination to sleep excessively, up to several hours longer than their usual amount. This is usually associated with some psychomotor retardation and exhaustion (see below). When coupled with increased appetite, mood reactivity, "leaden paralysis," and sensitivity to rejection, this variant is referred to as "atypical depression"—a historical term not reflective of the reality that these features are quite common (Zisook & Braff, 1985; Davidson et al., 1982).

In assessing hypersomnia, clinicians should also determine the extent to which depressed patients are actually sleeping more, rather than remaining in bed because they are amotivational, anergic, and psychologically "paralyzed." Yet another possibility is that patients are "actively" staying in bed as a way of avoiding demands that they can't meet, or as a means of shutting out some of the anguish and despair they experience when out of bed.

Assessing the clinical relevance of these variants of sleep disturbance focuses on the following questions: (1) Does the disturbance suggest an autonomous process? (2) Does the disturbance in and of itself account for other clinical features? (3) How is the person responding to the symptom and translating this experience into behavior? (4) Does the disturbance warrant intervention, and, if so, what kind?

Appetite Disturbances

Appetite disturbances are common, variable, and complicated. The prototypical change in major depression is the suppression of appetite—a loss of the drive to eat, a lack of interest in food, and at times even damping of the sense of taste. This is usually accompanied by substantial weight loss. At times people will eat normally despite this appetite suppression, out of habit or forced necessity, but it requires effort. This symptom is also common under acute duress, but when it is present on a continuing basis, it is a strong indication of the autonomy of the depression.

By contrast, a substantial number of individuals with major depression experience an increase in appetite and are inclined to gain weight. This symptom ("hyperphagia") may be much more difficult to define as specifically related to an autonomous depression, because of the large number of people caught in a vicious cycle of dysphoria-driven eating, weight gain, and subsequent low self-esteem contributing to a repetition of this behavior. Overlapping with this group are patients (mostly women) with diagnosed bulimia nervosa, who demonstrate frequent depressive symptoms and a high incidence of major depression. The relationship between bulimia nervosa and depression has yet to be clarified (Hadson et al., 1983). The overlap underscores the difficulty in determining the full relevance of a single depressive symptom in efforts to diagnose a depressive illness.

Diminished Energy and Fatigue

Persons with major depression feel depleted, exhausted, and drained of energy, both physically and emotionally. Every activity requires a huge expenditure of effort. The persons feel as though they are working against a gradient. At times this is clear from the patients' descriptions and the observations of family members, friends, and coworkers. However, other forces may mitigate against its potentially profound impact. Those who are unusually perfectionistic will appear at times frenetic in their efforts at completing tasks, which are made many times more difficult by their depression (with the accompanying lack of interest or pleasure inherent in the task, mental and physical exhaustion, and impaired cognition).

Psychomotor Agitation or Retardation

In depression, "nervous energy" is characterized by two seemingly antithetical states: one in which a person's "rheostat" is turned up (psychomotor agitation) and another in which it is turned down or off (psychomotor retardation). In agitated states, patients can appear physically shaky and describe a sense of physical trembling. Such states are usually associated with insomnia and anorexia in a depressive syndrome. The agitation is undirected and nonspecific, although it can become attached to a specific issue or idea and can become associated with endless focal rumination about guilt, loss, inadequacy, or suicide. This state needs to be differentiated from the anxiety symptoms characteristic of panic disorder, phobias, or generalized anxiety disorder. Although these latter symptoms are not integral characteristics of a depressive disorder, there is a very strong association between major depression and panic disorder (Grunhaus et al., 1994).

Whereas psychomotor agitation can be a feature of many functional psychiatric disorders (depression, anxiety disorders, dementias, psychoses), psychomotor retardation is more specific for major depression. Its presence in a depressive state should raise the clinician's index of suspicion for bipolarity, as retardation is often seen in the depressed state of a manic–depressive illness (Goodwin & Jamison, 1990). In some patients, states of agitation and retardation may alternate. For example, severely depressed persons may pace, pull at their hair, and wring their hands (agitation), while also thinking and talking slowly and delaying for long periods before initiating purposeful activity (retardation).

Anhedonia

Establishing the autonomy of depressive symptoms may be difficult. Mood, cognitive symptoms, and the other vegetative symptoms described to this point may seem like the products of immediate circumstances and stressors, exaggerations of long-standing personality variants, or reflections of existential truths. However, anhedonia—the lack of the capacity to experience pleasure—may be the most "pure" symptom of a depressive illness. Insofar as there is a very clear, identifiable "pleasure center" in the hypothalamus (the median forebrain bundle), its dysfunction is every bit as "biological" as sleep and appetite disturbances.

As is true of most biological functions, disruption of the pleasure function proceeds along a continuum. The loss or damping of pleasure or enjoyment can best be detected from an examination of the patient's own hierarchy of experiences, from the more mundane to the sublime. The most powerful experiences—intimacy with a child, the excitement of a changing career, or falling in love—may be retained or may "override" a faulty mechanism, leading to some pleasure and often a transient change in mood. More mundane experiences, on the other hand, may lose all their savor for the person. In some cases, the compulsions to gamble, go on spending sprees, or have affairs reflect desperate efforts to stimulate the capacity for enjoyment and escape the sense of emptiness that anhedonia creates.

Different neurophysiological mechanisms regulate sexual functioning. Central mechanisms seem to mediate and interpret pleasure, as well as the anticipation of pleasure. Depression is frequently accompanied by a loss of libido. However, since the peripheral sensory mechanisms are still intact, depressed people can usually still get physical pleasure from sexual activity; they simply do not desire or anticipate it.

In our opinion, anhedonia in a depressed patient is the most pathognomonic symptom of the disorder, and the one most likely to define the disorder as autonomous. Conversely, when an individual has retained the full capacity for enjoyment, we are reluctant to define a syndrome of clinical depression even if the person meets the other DSM-IV criteria for a major depressive episode. Under those circumstances, we are much more likely to view the other symptoms as fluid and reactive and to be more suspicious of their autonomy. Therefore, loss of interest or pleasure may be a more reliable indicator of clinical depression than dysphoria, especiallly in those individuals who are likely to minimize, deny, or not recognize depressed moods (e.g., the very young, the very old, and the medically ill).

COGNITIVE SYMPTOMS

Depression is characterized by disruptive changes in cognitive processes in two directions: (1) an impairment of functional efficiency (Bornstein et al., 1991), and (2) a distortion in interpretive processes (Beck et al., 1979).

Functional inefficiency can be a product of the impairment of several different elements. Depression can involve a slowing of mental processes or literal "mental retardation," which produces a form of pseudostupidity. Individuals may describe an inability to recall, interpret, calculate, or synthesize as a result of such slowing. Abstract thinking is impaired. Impaired concentration is a related symptom, at times associated with easy distractibility or more active processes involving intrusive thoughts or ideas as ruminations. As a result, there is an impairment in the retrieval of short-term memory and in the capacity for new learning (Bornstein et al., 1991).

In our experience, functional cognitive impairment is a late symptom, appearing after most other symptoms. It is also a symptom that often leads professional or other white-collar people into treatment. As other manifestations of depression appear at earlier stages, such people find themselves making adjustments—tolerating or compensating for changes in mood, sleep, energy, and so on. When symptoms disruptive to their occupational functioning occur, there is often a limit to what they can adjust before their careers and livelihoods are placed at risk.

By contrast, the distortive perceptions of depression usually make their appearance quite early in the course of an evolving mood disorder. There is a tendency to become more self-critical or deprecating; to feel guilty or responsible for problems in the world or one's own life; to become cynical about human nature or political processes; to be pessimistic or nihilistic about the future; and to despair of changing one's situation, with evolving helplessness, hopelessness, and suicidal ideation accompanying this despair. Changes in mood are often most readily evident in these accompanying inclinations.

The relationship of these cognitive distortions to mood is interesting and complex. The work of Beck (1976) has postulated a cognitive basis for mood disturbances: Negative thoughts can lead to a downward turn in mood, and, conversely, positive thoughts may improve mood. From a biological perspective, however, depressive illness causes a *primary* change in mood, which has the capacity to create distortions in thinking. However, once created, the negative cognitions in turn are likely to feed into a depressed mood in a more intense way. In other words, depression recruits negative thoughts about oneself, the world, and the future.

In order to appreciate the highly sensitive nature of these distorted cognitive perceptions in mood disturbances, it is important to understand them within a broader context of human experience. People almost universally view relationships in an ambivalent, if not continuum-like, manner. This includes their relationships to and observations about themselves, their friends and families, their cultures and religions, their countries, and humanity itself. Although people may believe themselves to be competent, confident, righteous, and caring, everyone has experienced feelings of inadequacy, insecurity, cruelty, and indifference at some time or other. These latent images are state-dependent; are associated with numerous potential dysphoric emotions; and are capable of being stimulated by and emerging with a variety of disruptive states, including depression.

Such a model is easily extended to other spheres of outlook or perspective. In the absence of depression, such distortions occur regularly; they are precipitated either primarily by another cognitive event (e.g., a TV show host reminds a viewer of his or her inferior looks or income) or by the evocation of a primary feeling state (e.g., a criticism by a supervisor leaves a worker feeling incompetent). In these circumstances, the potential for awakening, deepening, or generalizing the negative cognition is always present. Those people whose developmental experiences have led to a chronically impaired sense of self are inclined to do just that, and the momentary or temporary dysphoria created by such common experiences may be extended for them. Most people, however, naturally (consciously or unconsciously) set up a dialogue with themselves in which they argue successfully for their own adequacy and competency. A crucial element in the success of this dialogue, however, is the positive reinforcement of any view they may arrive at that helps balance things. To take the second example given above, the person who has been criticized by a supervisor is likely to seek out from experience other times when his or her efforts were appreciated or when he or she was praised for other abilities or was loved despite personal failings. In each of these memories there is a cognitive element of success, reinforced by an emotional experience of admiration or love. The potentially distressing and reinforcing cycle of negative thoughts and feelings is thus interrupted.

However, in the depressed person, the central mechanism for pleasure is not working, and the reinforcement of positive images does not occur; the balance and direction of cognitive perceptions are only shifted in a more negative direction. The depressed person is seeking a part of the "truth," but only the part that colors himself or herself, the world, and the future in its worst shades. These mechanisms are examined more fully in the next chapter.

SUICIDAL THOUGHTS

Clearly, the most dangerous of the cognitive distortions are those leading to feelings of helplessness and hopelessness. For the seriously depressed, such feelings make escape through suicide a logical extension of their experience. Regardless of the severity of a given depressive episode, people who have experienced depression over extended periods of time usually have some form of suicidal ideation. In the most common and mildest form, it may simply represent a wish to be free of the suffering inherent in depression. Evolution has probably provided all of us with a self-preservative drive, which does prevail for most depressed people most of the time; therefore, clinicians will frequently encounter depressed patients who may express a wish to be dead but "just can't do it" because of this drive. Other suicidal patients cling to life through their connections with loved ones, belief in God, fear of retribution, or other motivations (Schneidman et al., 1970).

It is critical, however, for clinicians to recognize that all of these life-saving mechanisms are relative and that depression and suffering, at a certain level of intensity and chronicity, can override them. Severe depression can and does have the capacity to overpower any other rational or instinctive force. All of these self-preservative processes are predicated upon the continuing effectiveness of the person's attachments to others or to life itself, and the maintenance of such attachments requires some demonstrable reinforcement to combat the forces of suffering—a function that is lost in severe depression. This is why major depression, among the illnesses known to humankind, is responsible for the highest rate of successful suicide throughout all age groups in all cultures. Even patients with terminal cancer rarely kill themselves in the absence of an accompanying major depression (Brown et al., 1986). Conversely, 10–15% of all people with major depression will ultimately commit suicide (Robins et al., 1959).

·4·

The Language of Depression

Although symptoms of depression are the defining features of clinical diagnosis, the effects of these symptoms on interpersonal behavior, identity, self-esteem, productive activities, and health constitute the "language" of depression—the way in which the depressed experience their world. The impact of depression on these all-encompassing dimensions of personality, functioning, and health provides us with an understanding of the profound disturbance and disability so often created by the disorder (Hirschfeld et al., 1983, 1989).

Recent data focusing on issues of quality of life indicate that patients with long-standing depression suffer as much (or more) and function as poorly as patients with heart disease, emphysema, arthritis, and other chronic illnesses (Wells et al., 1989; Agosti et al., 1991). Complicating this picture is the reality that the "language" of these other illnesses is largely somatic: the experience of physical pain, trouble breathing, and physical weakness. Although the illnesses usually have secondary effects on personality, these are often separable and definable, carrying little stigma beyond the sickness itself. On the other hand, the language of depression expresses itself in spheres of living that are often difficult to define and harder to separate from variations of normal functioning. At times this leaves the depressed unaware of what is causing their suffering and dysfunction, or, even when they are aware, struggling with a sense of inadequacy for not having a "legitimate" reason for their illness.

The capacity for depressive manifestations to appear "silently"—that is, without being announced—reflects two separate though often overlapping qualities. First, the emergence of depressive features can be quite insidious and gradual. White may not become blue overnight; instead, it may appear to change in subtle shades along each of the dimensions noted above. A sufferer may make a series of adjustments to these changes without registering that the changes have even occurred, until the impact on feeling and functioning becomes substantial. The second quality seems to be less an adaptational response than an innate property of depression, wherein the depressed person's perceptual and interpretative apparatuses are taken over by the depressed state. The individual becomes a "captive" and loses perspective, including the awareness that he or she is actually depressed; the person thus becomes incapable of recognizing that his or her distorted perceptions, interactions, and functioning are a result of "the depression talking." These qualities of the "silence" of depression—insidiousness and the loss of perspective— also result in the invisibility of the disorder to others.

Further complicating the potential for depression to cause maladaptive behavior is the tendency for people who are feeling dysphoric and misperceiving elements within their lives (themselves, their relationships, their work, etc.) to seize upon these misperceptions as valid and act upon them in an attempt to feel better. The hope of relief from their suffering creates a "moral imperative" that presses for action. When depression colors an individual's already ambivalent perceptions about a marriage or career, for example, the depressed person may seize upon such views as the impetus for change. This is seen as the solution to an existential dilemma; in reality, however, the person is unable to translate the language of depression accurately. Change may seem not only justified by the person's unbalanced and hypertrophied criticisms of the situation, but essential for his or her well-being. In a depressed state, there may be no questioning of whether there are other sides to decisions about leaving a marriage or job. The depressed person is unable to experience the positive elements of the relationship or the inherent satisfactions of the work, which may be overshadowed by the impact of depression. To appreciate fully the nature of such misperceptions, let us examine in detail the manifestations of depression in these and other dimensions.

EFFECTS ON
INTERPERSONAL RELATIONSHIPS

While irritability is no longer one of the diagnostic criteria for depression, it usually accompanies most depressed states. The depressed person may express this in the form of a harsh tone, a critical edge, or open hostility. Bitterness, cynicism, or misanthropy may poison relations with others. Even where there is an awareness of some positive features in an affectual relationship, this is overshadowed by criticism of the other person, as well as perceived criticism by the significant other (at times this may become a self-fulfilling prophecy or projection). Feeling dysphoric heightens one's sense of entitlement and lowers the capacity for consideration of others, as some patients are aware:

MARK: I have a tendency to push people away. I say really mean, insensitive things. I cannot seem to help myself. . . . After a while no one wants to be around me, because I am always in a bad mood.

A sense of personal vulnerability may cause patients to shut themselves off from relationships (see full case description in Chapter 8):

LINDA: A general lack of self-esteem has made it difficult for me to be open and honest with others, and as a result I have had only a few close friends. Particularly when depressed, I tend to withdraw and try to have as little interpersonal contact as possible. In part, this is an attempt to hide my inner feelings from others, coupled with great fear that the fraud that I am will be exposed.

Depressed persons also frequently manifest a form of resentment toward their primary caregivers, be they parents, spouses, or others. This seems to be a regression to a phenomenon that is normally seen in childhood: A parent is expected to bring relief to a child, regardless of the nature of the child's suffering (physical pain, unhappiness, frustration, or fear). The parent's limitations in the face of the child's omnipotent wishes give rise to anger. Very similar anger is frequently seen among patients with chronic illnesses (including depression) whose physicians and other caregivers cannot relieve their suffering. Among the depressed, the resentment may reflect not only the lack of hoped-for relief, but envy of the nonsuffering persons' "nonsuffering."

BOB: One way I can tell when I'm getting depressed again is the complete change in my feelings toward my wife, Lucille. Everything I love about her when I'm normal I hate in her when I'm depressed. It's palpable. She can see it in me. I'm ashamed of it. When I'm like this, the only way we can get along is by avoiding each other.

Such forces can work in both directions:

LYNN: I know I exhibited most of the classic signs of depression and must have been difficult to live with, but trying to explain that all I could do was survive from day to day, and that images of stabbing myself with a kitchen knife would sometimes fill my mind at night, only seemed to antagonize my husband. It was a cruel shock to feel betrayed by the person from whom I most expected and needed love and support. Unfortunately, his refusal to accept it protracted my depressive state and became the focus of all my suffering. I endured continual verbal hostility; I was labeled as "totally selfish," blamed for shirking my responsibilities, and accused of deceiving him and my doctor. Now that the depression has lifted, and I am returning to a normal state of mind, terrible resentment and an inability to forgive him are crippling our relationship emotionally and physically. While I accept that it was difficult for him to understand, I cannot forgive him for making no effort to even try.

Another feature of depression is social withdrawal, as noted above in the statement by Linda. This is a self-protective action that enables suffering persons to preserve their resources and to avoid interpersonal interactions, which may be perceived as too demanding. At an interpersonal level, such withdrawal may not create the degree of active conflict that irritability and resentment often do; however, significant others may not understand why this is occurring, and may misinterpret the behavior as criticism or rejection of them. Linda elaborated further on her withdrawal:

LINDA: I fear that my desire for solitude and unreasonable expectations have at times made me a poor mother and wife. Although when depressed I would desperately want to flee and hide, a strong sense of obligation and guilt would compel me to try to engage in the interactions expected of me. This was not an easy task, particularly with respect to my relationship with my husband. My inability to derive pleasure from any activity, including sex, obviously put a serious strain on our marriage. Furthermore, my withdrawal, irritability, and lack of enjoyment of life in general would send the inappropriate message that I no longer cared for the people who meant the most to me.

Another patient noted the link between withdrawal and anger:

JACK: My lover has borne the brunt of my anger at my unhappiness. I have expected him to empathize with my feelings, but I never feel that he really understands how I feel. That makes me think there is a great emotional distance between us. To bridge the gap, I either withdraw in order to punish him, or I start to nag and criticize, hoping to get a response. He invariably gets angry and I invariably hate myself. Then we reconcile, and the next day the cycle starts over again.

The maintenance of a good marriage or similar relationship usually requires effort, patience, understanding, personal strength, a sense of balance, and a sense of humor. Elements of depression mitigate against all of these factors. The depressed person feels depleted of energy and interest in working on the relationship. He or she lacks the resilience and flexibility necessary to struggle through the inevitable conflicts of such a relationship; the person simply cannot tolerate being "hassled" and either withdraws or becomes hostile. He or she seems unable to persevere in the face of distress. There is also a loss of perspective about the relationship, with distortions about the person's own self-worth, adequacy, lovability, or entitlement to happiness on the one hand, and the emptiness, meaninglessness, or dissatisfaction of the relationship on the other.

As noted earlier, the dissatisfaction becomes particularly sharp in cases where mood changes exacerbate areas of conflict and criticism that were previously balanced by other qualities. Now the positive qualities seem to disappear and the negative ones are hugely magnified. Or the same qualities are seen in the light of the prevailing mood: the spouse or partner who was seen as stable and thoughtful is now "boring"; the generous one is now wasteful; the reserved one is withholding; the humorous one is sarcastic and hurtful. Table 4.1 shows how those and other characteristics are distorted by depression. One can easily extrapolate from these examples to see how an almost inexhaustible number of qualities may be affected. Furthermore, in the throes of depression, bombarded by so many forms of emotional suffering and negativity, a depressed spouse or partner often becomes self-centered, focused on his or her personal anguish. Under these circumstances, there is a loss of the capacity for consideration and empathy for the other person, which contributes further to the deterioration of the relationship.

Beyond the regressive transformation of negotiating and coping skills within relationships, the depressed bring yet another potentially destructive element to relationships—the power of their moods.

BERNICE: It has limited my friendships to extremely loyal individuals who can handle my mood swings.

FRAN: I want to avoid subjecting my family and friends to my state of depression. I don't want to make them have to deal with the stress of being with someone so down.

TABLE 4.1. Depressive Distortions of a Partner's Attributes

Partner's "normal" attribute	Distorted attribute
Humor	Cruelty
Generosity	Wastefulness
Frugality	Withholding
Reserve	Lack of feeling
Stability	Dullness
Confidence	Arrogance
Concern	Intrusiveness
Consideration	Weakness
Affection	Dependency

Patients are often quite aware of the impact that their negative moods can have on others. If their friends or family members are supportive and empathic, they will probably suffer from their exposure to the persistent, sustained depressive states.

JACK: I nearly lost a good friend because her depression ended and mine didn't. . . . It was clear that she was no longer as desperately unhappy and I remained "stuck." We couldn't relate to each other any longer.

Even when others are willing and strong enough to tolerate and endure this exposure for brief periods, many depressed persons are reluctant to inflict themselves on these others. There is usually some limit to the capacity of others, including parents and spouses, to bear up under the oppressive weight of depression. This is heightened when the mood is accompanied by sustained self-deprecation, pessimism, and (in the extreme) hopelessness and suicidal preoccupation. Nondepressed persons' sense of helplessness in the face of all this can lead them to withdraw their support, especially when they are themselves somewhat rigid, narcissistic, or controlling and need to see the effectiveness of their own contact or input. Such people may have difficulty appreciating that the depressed persons' suffering is not directed at them.

One patient, Karen, was able to define her relationships on the basis of the other persons' responses to her:

KAREN: To my surprise, there are also people who are only friendly during a crisis. They call to see how I'm doing, do errands for me, and so on. But when I get better, the interest ceases. I suppose they move on to some other "project." I have a few friends who have stuck with me through good times and bad, who quietly notice how I'm doing and make adjustments without fanfare. They are persistent in inviting me to do whatever I feel up to—if they ask me to go to a restaurant for dinner and I balk, they suggest bringing a take-out meal to the house. These are the most valued friends, for they make me feel that they care about me personally. They don't consider me to be an extra burden, even though befriending a depressed person is sometimes very hard work.

Another group of depressed patients will be inclined to intensify their sense of interpersonal neediness, rejection sensitivity, and entitlement; in their desperation, they experience some actual loosening of their boundaries. These phenomena put another kind of pressure on relationships: Significant others often feel overwhelmed by these demands for support and intimacy, especially when they represent a substantial departure from the depressed persons' usual way of being.

Under usual circumstances, many marriages or similar relationships survive through periods of prolonged conflict and distress by achieving some positive balance through sexual intimacy. Here again, the effects of depression often make this impossible. The depressed partner's libido may be diminished or absent. Pleasure in sexual relations may be impeded or simply avoided. Sexual dysfunction in performance is common. The nondepressed partner may feel hurt and rejected. The relationship is thrown still further out of balance.

Depression takes a toll on relationships even under the most ideal of circumstances. Let us assume that the depressed person shows his or her suffering at those times when the partner is most receptive, supportive, and strong, and at other times finds ways to contain them to protect the other person; let us also assume that the nondepressed partner has an enormous capacity for empathy, a full appreciation for the struggles of the depressed person, and a willingness to do whatever is necessary to sustain the relationship and help the depressed person. Even under such circumstances as these, there is a great weight to bear and periods when the relationship will falter. This is especially true when depression becomes chronic and there is a substantial and continuous change in the personality of the depressed person. Because of this change, the chronic suffering experienced in the relationship, or the persistence of suicidal crises, the nondepressed partner may begin to reconsider his or her commitment.

In the case of a threat posed by a depressed partner to a marriage or relationship, the perception that the inherent nature of the relationship is poor and that a change will bring relief of such an "existential" crisis is the greatest risk. As noted earlier, this view assumes that the depressed person has lost perspective, cannot see the state-dependent regressive changes wrought by the depression (i.e., is a "captive" of the state), and feels a *moral imperative* to act in a way that he or she believes will improve matters. This is an extremely difficult situation for a clinician to assess, because of the impact of depression on the depressed person's perceptions and the fact that this may be the complaint at the point of clinical presentation, before the clinician has had time for any independent assessment of the relationship. For all of these reasons, a chief complaint of relationship problems should at least raise the suspicion of depression as a significant contributing factor or primary issue.

Lest the reader be left with the impression that there are only destructive or maladaptive consequences for the relationships of the depressed, it must be appreciated that some good can arise from suffering and from the efforts of the depressed and their loved ones to cope with it:

LYNN: On the brighter side, I was able to heal a relationship that for most of my life has been remote and painful. I have never felt close to or loved by my father. The concern he showed and the effort he made to understand what I was experiencing was a total surprise.

MARCIA: The depression has strengthened my family relationships in many ways. It forced us to discuss the family history of depression, and I also became dependent on them for the first time in years. I lived with my parents for a summer when I reached a point where I was unable to work.

I have come to view my close friendships differently. I was amazed to find out how much I could actually count on them. On the other hand, it continues to amaze me that most people do not want to hear about the reality of depression.

EFFECTS ON PRODUCTIVE CAPACITIES

As Chapter 3 has described, the symptoms of depression include changes in formal cognitive processes, cognitive distortions, interpersonal problems, vegetative symptoms, motivational impediments, and diminished coping skills. In most circumstances, these areas of dysfunction interact in various ways to create a complex picture of compromised functional and productive capacities (Mintz et al., 1992).

As a manifestation of anhedonia, the depressed person's sense of enjoyment and satisfaction with his or her job or career is diminished or absent, undermining the motivation for work. At the same time, the person's pessimism and self-deprecation may lead to greater devaluation of the work itself, as well as to the view that he or she is incapable of doing it well, or at least to doubts about capability. The person may go on to develop questions about his or her motives for pursuing the present job or career in the first place, and, in keeping with the general tone of the mood, very critical interpretations of these motives.

KAREN: I took great pride in my professional accomplishments, feeling that I had chosen an academic career where I could make a real contribution without sacrificing my principles. But when I got depressed, I saw my job as doing inconsequential paperwork without sacrificing my lifestyle. . . . I once thought I would make a difference in the world, molding public policy or leading a revolution or helping the poor. Instead, I find myself too overwhelmed to even go to a store.

When formal cognitive difficulties appear (impaired concentration and short-term memory, indecision, distractibility, intrusive ruminations, and impaired capacity for learning), these contribute not only to the depressed person's perception but to a certain reality-based view of his or her inadequacy. Usually, such difficulties are perceived not as time-limited or state-dependent, but as indicating the "true" nature of the person's abilities, in contrast to the more "illusory" state of being when the person is feeling and functioning well.

FRAN: Depression and frustration and anger all brought my functioning at work finally to a complete stop. My brain simply stopped processing incoming data. I couldn't read a memo and have understanding of concepts because I couldn't remember what I'd read. Communicating with others left me exhausted, angry, not understanding why it all seemed so blocked and difficult.

LYNN: I couldn't concentrate on one task for longer than a couple of minutes. I found myself forgetting who I had talked to and where I had left things. Unable even to use a calculator, I would count on my fingers and still get basic arithmetic wrong.

Interpersonal factors complicate such situations because of depressed persons' inclination toward irritability or withdrawal, lack of resilience in dealing with others, and limited capacity to persevere in the face of these pressures. If one adds to this a lack of sleep or fatigue, it is easy to see how impaired a depressed person may become.

People suffering from depression find themselves without the physical and mental energy to participate in their work in more efficient ways. Such people often describe carrying out their roles and jobs as "automatons," with minimal involvement in the task and only the most marginal performance. This can continue for extended periods, with only limited awareness on the part of coworkers and employers. This is especially true in circumstances where aspects of a job are repetitive or rote, where creativity is only occasionally demanded, where a depressed individual has much autonomy or is self-employed, or where a depressed supervisor has effective help through delegation of responsibilities. However these mitigating factors may operate, those with depression often learn that they can keep colleagues and supervisors "in the dark" for extended periods. Most jobs have some margin of error or safety built into them that accommodates "down time" or allows for inadequate performance when an individual is not efficient. In other circumstances, depressed individuals' supervisors or colleagues are aware of the problem and can support them in their compromised functioning. This is usually tolerable for short periods of time before a supportive network seeks some relief (e.g., a supervisor asks a depressed worker to take some kind of disability leave). Of course, there are also many situations in which there is little tolerance for depressed persons' limitations; this reinforces the continued efforts to hide such difficulties and compensate for them in whatever ways are possible.

KAREN: I felt like the work was incredibly trivial, wondering what difference could it possibly make in the real world if the work never got done.

Previously I took great pride in my professional accomplishments, but then I lost interest completely. My error rate went up; my productivity went down. Instead of enjoying the intellectual challenge of my work, I found myself sticking things on a "problem" shelf if they were not perfectly routine (and sometimes even the routine seemed problematic). I lost the ability to set priorities, and so I spent a lot of time on unimportant things, meaning other things just didn't get done. I could still carry out familiar tasks and deal with broad concepts, but learning new skills or doing something really detailed (like computer programming) was impossible.

LINDA: My first major episode of depression occurred at age 18, during the fall semester of my freshman year of college. Because I placed out of introductory biology and calculus, my course load of advanced calculus, vertebrate zoology, advanced Russian, and English literature placed demands on me that even without depression would have strained my intellectual capabilities. I slept little at night and awoke early each morning with dread for the day ahead. Although my ability to concentrate and retain new material was markedly diminished, my level of persistence and perseverance increased. With a sense of self that was predicated on achievement, the fear of failure became the compelling force that drove me to study and work long hours, albeit at greatly reduced efficiency. Life held no pleasure other than the relief late at night that another day had ended. By sheer determination I passed my courses that semester, and when the depression began to lift during the second semester, I was again able to derive satisfaction from my studies and other activities.

Depression recurred while I was a graduate student and has periodically made its appearance during my adult years. As a mother, wife, and professional woman with a career that demands 60- to 70-hour weeks, I have found that my life has had little tolerance for the dysfunction resulting from these depressive episodes. Fortunately, my job allows me to be relatively independent, with no one monitoring my activities on an hourly or daily basis. Thus at work, I have been able to compensate for the periods of impaired function by working longer hours both during the depression and immediately afterwards. The fear of failure that characterized my student experience has maintained its dominant position, thereby ensuring that the level of persistence and perseverance would increase as my capacity to perform diminished. The cost, however, has been substantial. During the periods of depression, so much of my energy would be consumed by laboring long hours and hiding the inner turmoil from my colleagues that I had little left for my children or husband. Household decisions and tasks that normally could be accomplished with ease became Sisyphean. And yet my sense of responsibility and guilt over shortchanging the people who meant the most to me provided a strong impetus for at least trying to continue to function. In many ways during these periods, my actions became automated as the inner self that was in pain tried to withdraw and the outer shell took over. I suspect that much of the motivation for this continued function was generated from the fear that if I succumbed to the urge to withdraw completely, my true self—the one that I believed to be a failure and incompetent—would be fully exposed for all to see.

Depression in the workplace is often experienced as "burnout." This term has come to describe the increased stress and distress that many individuals encounter in the workplace. Certainly, many factors can contribute to the sense that one's work is "too much." All work has inherently difficult aspects, whether these are mental, physical, or emotional. (That's why it's called "work.") People may feel harassed from above or below, or they may feel unappreciated or underpaid. The demands of a job or career may conflict with an individual's need for time or emotional energy for other relationships or for relaxation. Economic hardships may push a person toward work that is unsatisfying or demeaning. All of these issues suggest that qualities of the workplace or of a specific job are the focus most relevant to the experience of "burnout." However, if one considers the manifestations of depression in the workplace, one can see that much of what is described as "burnout" may reflect aspects of the mood disorder.

The examples with which we are most familiar occur in our own workplace—that is, among mental health workers. In this setting, the most common form of burnout is related to the inherent stresses of working with people who are suffering. Laypeople often comment that they don't know how therapists can deal with so much anguish, turmoil, and complaining on a daily basis. On the other hand, people are drawn into the helping professions for many positive reasons. These include the capacity for empathy, a natural curiosity about others, a need to help, the pleasure of being important to others, and the self-enrichment resulting from the intimacy that such work fosters. The therapeutic enterprise is a stimulating and enriching experience, all the more so when it is successful. It may be quite "weighty" as well, in terms of helping others bear the burdens of their suffering. Empathy exacts a toll from therapists, but skilled therapists develop some clinical distance to limit such effects. Over the years, there may be some normal erosion of enthusiasm and optimism, a "jading" that arises from seeing the limitations of therapeutic efforts. Or a greater detachment may develop—one that both protects therapists and lessens the effective and rewarding aspects of emotional contact. In extreme cases, therapists may become demoralized about the never-ending flood of human misery. Although these manifestations of burnout may reflect "normal" processes, they may also be part of the language of depression.

In this setting, how does depression manifest itself? Most importantly, the burden of patients' suffering becomes greater. Because of the prevailing mood of depressed helpers, they are likely to have a more intense empathic response: The therapists resonate more profoundly with themes of depression and have more difficulty extricating themselves from this state. They are also less likely to mobilize those intellectual skills that are necessary for both making clinical decisions and maintaining appropriate distance. Some therapists' boundaries become more fluid when they are depressed, forcing them to withdraw emotionally just to protect themselves. In contrast to the sense of mastery and satisfaction that accompanies controlled regressions, depressed therapists are likely to feel overwhelmed, doubting, or incompetent in their efforts. Therapeutic optimism or realism turns to pessimism or nihilism in their individual efforts, as well as their views about their field as a whole. Under siege from their internal state, and feeling more vulnerable because of it, therapists may become intolerant of their patients or begin to misconstrue patients' behavior as manipulative and demeaning, even if they previously saw the same behavior as desperate but maladaptive (views that were "kinder" and less self-directed). Under the influence of depression, therapists may begin to reexamine and reinterpret their prior motives for their work in critical and destructive ways, emphasizing the self-serving rather than the altruistic. They may see themselves as people who want to control and manipulate others rather than help them; as voyeuristic in contrast to curious and interested; as nurturing their own dependency and narcissism; and, in response to their protective detachment, as uncaring, unfeeling persons just doing a job.

If all of these forces are operating *without perspective*—without the recognition that this is "depression talking," and that this state is time-limited and state-dependent—depressed therapists may perceive their state as a career-related existential crisis whose solution is change. Enough elements within this configuration parallel "normal" burnout that change may come to seem a "moral imperative" for depressed helpers. Unless they recognize the numerous elements of depression that are manifesting themselves not only in their work but in other aspects of their lives, they may see these as messages telling them to quit.

IMPACT ON IDENTITY AND SELF-ESTEEM

Several patients have described vivid images of themselves when depressed:

BARBARA: I'm sitting in a corner with my shoulders slouched forward and my head down. I am feeling a lot of shame. I am wearing a black scarf. . . . I have on a T-shirt with a big "D" on it. There are several plants around me that are dead. I am wearing rubber boots that come up to my knees—

since there are puddles of water around me from all the crying and weeping I've been doing. There is a clock on the wall—the face is cracked and "time has stopped." I have surface and deeper wounds on my arms, since I "emotionally" wound very easily when depressed. My mind isn't working—there are Scrabble letters on the floor—I can't unscramble them to make any words. At times I feel like I'm "burning up" with rage, because I feel angry about how this disease has affected me, so at times it feels like fire is coming out of my mouth. I have a lock on the phone. I don't want to talk to anyone.

DANIEL: Every morning when I wake, I ask myself: Who am I? Why should I get out of bed? For what purpose? My reality during my waking hours seems to be so much different than others that I have no sense of purpose. If I died today, who would notice? Who would care? Why?

BERNICE: My most severe depressions make my self-esteem and identity so meaningless that I literally wish to die. Any degree of depression makes me feel isolated from what I perceive as all the "normal" people's happy lives. My failures are prominent in my thoughts. . . . I really feel at those moments of depression that my negative physical traits are real and permanent. I blame myself for not having the willpower to do things that will make me feel better. In truth, I don't believe anything would make me feel better, including winning the lottery, being asked out by a handsome prince, or being elected president of something.

ANN: I often feel that I will never be all right—never have a "normal" life. No matter how much I accomplish, it is never enough.

JACK: All my life I have felt inadequate, personally responsible for my depression, helpless, weak, worthless, very needy, out of control, and lacking in moral fiber. Everything I have ever achieved or tried to achieve was motivated by a desire to boost my self-esteem and identity. As the depression has worsened, I have grown increasingly desperate because nothing I can achieve makes me feel better about myself. Then life starts feeling hopeless.

We have already alluded to a number of the ways in which depression distorts how people think about others, their work, and themselves. Central to our understanding of the distortions of self-concept that occur in depressive states is the recognition of self-concept as a dynamic, slowly evolving process. Certain universal themes with myriad variations are played out in the lives of all people. If people develop in the most adaptive and healthy ways, they arrive at views about themselves and about the world that are balanced, but preponderantly positive. Such healthy persons might be described as confidently humble, sensitively assertive, optimistically realistic, autonomously interdependent, capably learning, masterfully vulnerable, and so on. Regardless of the most ideal or mature state or view at which such persons arrive, their journey has included experiences of failure, rejection, abuse, and inadequacy; feelings of being overwhelmed and out of control; and at least moments of grief, helplessness, and despair. In healthy people, these latent negative states and their accompanying negative self-images are usually overshadowed by positive states—images of themselves and the world that are augmented by suppression, repression, and other compensatory mechanisms. Such people may be able to remember or reexperience latent negative states and images through therapeutic regression; however, if given a choice, most of them would choose to ignore or actively avoid such experiences. Depression offers no choice: It *actively recruits* negative states.

Although it is unclear why such phenomena occur, one explanation comes from the theory of state-dependent learning: Associational pathways (memories, images) are stimulated by affective states similar to those in which the experience first occurred. This theory provides a neurophysiological basis for Freud's (1915/1957) ideas on free association. It also suggests that a crucial element in our understanding of the language of depression is the *artifactual* nature of many of depression's effects on identity and self-esteem. What do we mean by this?

Three interactive forces in depression lead to pessimism and negative self-images: (1) the dynamic and developmental themes, both idiosyncratic and universal; (2) the reality-based functional impairment; and (3) the driving force of the negative affective state. Of these three concurrent processes, the second and third are direct consequences of depression, and the third is by far the greatest contributor to the formation of negative self-images. Let us consider the three processes separately.

To begin with the second process mentioned above, depressed persons' views of themselves and the world can be profoundly influenced by their "correct" observations of their areas of impairment. They will see themselves as less flexible and resilient, slower, less adequate, more dependent but less socially capable, less intelligent, more dissatisfied and frustrated, less tolerant, and less confident about themselves. These are reality-based views; however, these particular aspects of "reality" are shaped by the effects of the depression.

Developmental and dynamic contributions to self-regressions also determine the quality or character of such states. However, confusion often occurs when clinicians mistakenly place inordinate emphasis on the particular dynamic issues reflected in these regressions. As comedian Myron Cohen once replied, when asked by an irate husband why he was hiding in the man's wife's closet, "Everybody's got to be some-place." Similarly, every depressive episode occurs in the context of the idiosyncratic developmental issues of that person's life at that moment. Whether the person is struggling with issues of separation and individu-ation, intimacy with others, career development, or changes connected with aging, these issues will manifest themselves in the regressive schemes of the depressed person. For example, all people struggle internally with processes of aging. The occurrence of depression at that time may not be a product of any aspect of those processes or the individual's struggle with them; however, when depression is superimposed on such a ma-trix, it will certainly intensify the sufferer's negative self-concepts and future orientation—probably in the direction of his or her feeling more dependent and less adequate, and emphasizing personal deterioration and pessimism, even though continued personal growth and optimism may have previously dominated.

Aside from the idiosyncratic dynamic or developmental contribu-tion, there is also a universal dynamic that operates in shaping such self-regressions. By the term "universal dynamic," we mean the predictable and almost stereotypical regressive response to a specific area of regres-sion that has been precipitated by the depression. Self-conceptual dis-tortions will reflect the dynamic themes of dysfunction. Thus, when depression leads to irritability, social withdrawal, or interpersonal hyper-sensitivity, self-concepts will regress in the direction of the individual's sense of isolation, alienation, social incompetency, or incapacity for in-timacy. When work function is impaired, self-concepts will gravitate to perceptions of being inept, a failure, overly dependent on others, or the like. Although in each of these examples other historical and dynamic factors will interact further with these areas of dysfunction to create the final picture, the primary shaping force, aside from the depression itself, is the specific dysfunction.

LINDA: When depressed I view myself as a total failure, as an individual who has not earned the right to exist. I see my research and publications as worthless, my interactions with my children and husband as ineffectual and detrimental to their well-being, and my service to the community as non-descript. I feel that I am no more than an empty shell with no identity and nothing inside of any substance. Most of all, I become convinced that I am a fraud and have somehow tricked my colleagues into promoting me and my husband and children into loving me. Great fear overwhelms me that the tidal wave of truth will soon engulf me. I also have a sense of being in a dark, deep hole, and alternately wish that the hole would completely close or that I could find my way out to the light. Yet my sense of hopelessness and failure intensify the longer I stay in the hole, as I realize that only through my own efforts will I be able to climb out.

MARCIA: I became convinced that I was a burden on other people. This did not allow me to maintain my sense of independence that I had worked so hard to achieve since I was very young. I think this contributed greatly to the suicidal feelings I had for many months.

When the prevailing mood of depression interacts with the reality-based impairment and the developmental and dynamic forces that are either preexisting or reactive, the results can be overwhelming and devastating. The regression in self-concept (both current and retroactive), and in belief systems about the world and the future, can become all-consuming. Most significantly, it can lead to the existential crisis that is irreversible and lethal—suicide. Depressed persons who see themselves as trapped in unrelenting suffering without hope are quite likely to experience at least the wish to be relieved of such suffering. The risk of suicide is greatest when an individual is truly a "captive" of the depression—unable to recognize the time-limited, state-dependent, artifactual nature of this experience. Under these circumstances, the "moral imperative" can be suicide.

HEALTH CONSEQUENCES

People who are depressed have shorter lives than the nondepressed, even if they do not commit suicide; they also have more comorbidity in terms of other medical problems than the nondepressed (Wells et al., 1989). Because there are numerous medical causes of depression, it is crucial that every depressed patient be evaluated to make sure that there is no endocrine, neurological, toxicological, infectious, pharmacological, or other medical reason for its appearance. The health consequences of depression can be considered from three perspectives: (1) the inherent vegetative dysfunctions of depression; (2) health consequences associated with the biological changes that accompany depression, and (3) the health consequences of the behavioral changes of depression. Furthermore, the negative effects of depression upon health can aggravate or contribute to already existing dysfunction in relationships, work, and self-concept.

Both the immediate and the long-term effects of the vegetative symptoms of depression are self-defining. Most people would agree that it is unhealthy to lose sleep or to sleep excessively; not to eat or to eat excessively; to be weak, tired, depleted, and immobilized, or, conversely, to be continually agitated, anxious, worried, or guilty. In other words, such symptoms themselves represent poor health.

There are numerous other somatic symptoms and disorders associated with depression, including gastrointestinal, gynecological/urological/sexual, cardiovascular, endocrinological, neurological, musculoskeletal, and immune system disturbances (Schulberg et al., 1987; Pies, 1994). The mechanisms for these disturbances are not well understood, but they are thought to be associated with changes in the hypothalamic and pituitary functions that regulate processes in the autonomic nervous system, as well as with changes in the adrenal medullary regulation of stress and its interaction with the immune system. Whatever the mechanisms involved, depressed patients are quite vulnerable to the development of other illnesses.

The negative health consequences described above are primarily biological phenomena—direct or indirect products of the physiological processes that are the underpinnings of depression. Many of these dovetail with the results of changing behaviors, which also contribute to compromised health. Depression undermines many normal and habitual behaviors that are deemed health-promoting. The first of these is physical activity. Clearly, a modicum of exercise contributes to health; in depressed persons, however, the inclination to exercise is usually compromised by fatigue and slowing, as well as by the lack of energy, interest, and sustained motivation necessary to pursue regular physical activity. Even when depressed individuals know that walking or running improves their mood substantially, they find it hard to get started or to persevere with such activity.

Depression also wreaks havoc with people's weight. Patients who lose interest in food may require much encouragement or the remnants of their discipline to eat enough to sustain themselves. Others find that dysphoria pushes them to seek out food in order to comfort themselves or to satisfy cravings. They may struggle with the added weight, depleted by the depression of their energy and willpower, and feeling entitled by their suffering to soothe themselves by any means possible. This frame of mind can lead not only to substantial overeating, but to overindulgence in or abuse of drugs, alcohol, and tobacco, as well as to indiscriminate or risky sexual activity.

These "unhealthy" behaviors can further complicate or aggravate already existing dysfunction in interpersonal, productive, and/or self-perceptual spheres. This is especially true for issues of self-perception: Depressed people frequently see indulgence and lack of control as signs of personal or moral weakness, inadequacy, and failure. For those whose self-esteem may be particularly tied to their appearance, problems with food may be especially disturbing and reinforcing of their worst self-perceptions.

DEVELOPMENTAL CONSEQUENCES

Studies of the epidemiology and natural history of depression have greatly increased our understanding of how the disorder develops. In particular, it has increased our appreciation of how early in life depression appears (Kovacs et al., 1994) and how frequently it evolves into a chronic disorder (Keller et al., 1984). In regard to the latter point, although there are still many people who suffer intermittent episodes, those who have chronic forms of depression have come to utilize an increasing amount of professional help. This has come about as a result of an increasing awareness of the problem, both professionally and through public educational efforts, better diagnostic skills, and an expansion of both pharmacological and psychotherapeutic approaches. The effects of chronic depression are discussed further below.

Let us now consider the former point—the language of depression among the very young. What is the impact of depression when it invades the life of a child? Although our understanding of depression in childhood is that the essential elements are similar to those occurring in adults, three distinguishing features of childhood depression make it potentially more devastating. The first of these differences is the "captivity" of the child, especially the latency or prelatency child. When adults become depressed, they are often compromised in their capacity to retain perspective—to recognize that there is something different, that the phenomena they are experiencing are as a result of an altered state, that they are "not themselves." Even when they have been consumed by the depression, once it passes there is almost always some recognition of what has occurred and some capacity to differentiate that experience from "normal." Children are much more vulnerable to becoming "lost" in their depressions. They have neither the life experience or at times the cognitive capacities to make such distinctions; what they are going through is their reality. Just as abused children love their parents and often accept the abuse as the normal course of events, children who have been immersed in depression come to believe that this experience is normal, and in a cruel fashion it *can* become "normal" for them.

Regardless of whether a person is cognitively and emotionally a "captive" of the depressed state, it is inherently unpleasant and counterproductive. People with depression do try to fight against it and its effects, except in the most severe forms of depression, where people are physically and emotionally paralyzed. Again, children are at a greater disadvantage in this respect, because they lack the internal resources and developmental strengths of adults. They are less able to tolerate painful affects, to utilize hard-won skills in mastering their relationships, or to struggle with depression's assaults on their functional capacities and self-concepts.

The third disadvantage of childhood depression (and potentially its most devastating) is that through its powerful and immediate effects upon crucial areas of personality functioning, the development of these areas is changed. Children who lack energy, who can't enjoy, who can't concentrate, who are sullen and withdrawn, who are self-critical, and who have no confidence—that is, children who are depressed—will not explore, play, learn, develop interpersonal skills, or believe in the value or goodness of life, people, or themselves. When depressive episodes occur with any frequency, or depression is continuous, the developmental arrest or maladaptive divergence can be profound. Although self-preservative instincts keep people alive, their motivations to accomplish goals and find satisfaction are predicated upon intact biological systems that allow them to experience and anticipate pleasure. When these mechanisms malfunction in adults, beliefs and motivational systems may be compromised and distorted. Usually, however, they are strong enough to weather all but the worst depressions, and the systems are relatively intact when the depression passes. Children do not have such structures as firmly in place and are made more vulnerable by their absence at the moment. Furthermore, the structures of their futures (since some structure is always present) are likely to be ill suited for healthy living. Such children are likely to grow up with expectations of unhappiness, feelings of self-deprecation, and cynicism or pessimism about the world.

Thus, depression is no less a developmental trauma than abuse, neglect, separation, or death. In the evolution of self-concept, it may be worse. Although children have an inclination to feel responsible for whatever befalls them, in instances where there may have been "real" external culprits, some children can come to see themselves as genuine victims. This may mitigate against the view that they are the causes of their own suffering. By contrast, no child ever perceives himself or herself as the victim of depression. As disruptive as it may be, it is a fortunate outcome for depressed children to be able to experience resentment toward and to blame parents or culpable others for their misery. At least it affords them some personal protection, and sympathetic parents are more likely to be able to cope with such attacks from the children than the children are if they are attacking themselves.

Although the impact of depression upon personality is the most striking in observations of child development, parallel issues must be considered among those adults whose depressions have become chronic and continuous. We have already examined the myriad forms of regression manifested by depressed adults in areas of interpersonal, productive, and self-conceptual functioning; however, we have considered these regressions as time-limited and state-dependent. What are the consequences of chronic depression for those who suffer from it? What is the impact of chronic depression on adult development? In such circumstances, extrapolation from the short-term to the long-term effects yields a picture of significant deterioration in each area of functioning. Relationships are undermined as a depressed adult's social isolation increases. Progressive work disability changes the depressed person's career status from temporary disability with a job waiting to unemployability because of continuing absences from the workplace and the increasing self-perception of incapacity. With chronicity, the depressed person's perception of "not being myself" evolves into a belief that "this is what I am"—a view without remission or hope. The person may become emotionally constricted to shut out suffering, despair, or the continuing struggle with suicide. Whatever positive beliefs about the self or the world that the person may have held are gradually and often completely eroded. Over time, in short, the chronically depressed do become different people.

DEPRESSION IN "MORE HEALTHY" AND "LESS HEALTHY" PERSONALITIES

The apparent paradox of defining a person as a "healthy depressive" reflects two critical aspects of our integrative biological approach. The first is that fundamental elements of personality are separable from the elements of depression. This is clearly complicated by the numerous interactions between personality and symptomatic disorders that we have been describing. The "figure–ground" distinction has so many overlapping elements that a clinician would have to adopt this perspective even to begin to separate them in many instances. This task of separation is easier to demonstrate by contrasting depressed individuals whose premorbid personalities are at the "more healthy" end of a continuum with ones whose personalities are at the "less healthy" end. Second, the concept of a "healthy depressive" underscores the differences between our model and traditional models that attribute symptomatic illness to "unhealthy" dimensions of personality (i.e., unresolved conflicts, developmental deficits, and ineffective defense mechanisms).

What is a healthy personality? Recognizing that "healthy" does not mean "perfect," we classify personality variables within several different domains as either "relatively healthy/adaptive" or "relatively unhealthy/

maladaptive" in Table 4.2. The personality characteristics within these two categories represent the stable and usual configurations of qualities that make up premorbid personalities. Using this scheme, let us now consider the impact of depression upon individuals at each end of the "adaptive–maladaptive" continuum, to emphasize the considerable differences in their final clinical pictures. We also examine the variable manifestations of depression by looking at different degrees of the disorder as they are *superimposed* on such personality structures. As depression progresses from its mild to moderate to severe degrees of intensity, more symptoms are recruited; they worsen; and they are translated into different and increasingly severe forms of regression in relationships, work, identity, and coping.

Depression in "More Healthy" Personalities

When depression begins to assert itself in relatively healthy persons, its earliest manifestations may be mild changes in mood, energy, or capacity for pleasure. Although the persons may notice these changes, they may have no impact or only very subtle impact in other spheres; perhaps the persons feel diminished enthusiasm about work, have a little more difficulty getting started in the morning, seem a bit less gregarious, or are less likely to exercise. At the same time, these persons may not want to appear as if they are having any problems, and want to be as productive and appear to others to be as much "in control" as usual. Such persons have the internal resources to compensate for these changes, and through additional efforts are able to push themselves to maintain high levels of functioning.

As depression worsens, perhaps affecting sleep and leading to greater depressed mood, anergy, and anhedonia, these persons find that some perseverance is necessary to maintain functioning. Fortunately, they have adequate reservoirs of trust, security, and intimacy to contain their feelings of annoyance with their spouses or partners. They can maintain smiles on their faces to avoid being a burden on others. Their self-esteem is strong enough to give them a wide margin of safety when they are bombarded by self-doubts and intermittent self-driven assaults. Their views on how people should behave stay firm, even though they may feel apathetic and demoralized by their depression. In other words, healthy people can tolerate a significant amount of depression without obvious decompensation in personality functioning, even though they are suffering considerably. The expenditure of effort may be enormous, but their internal resources, margins of safety, intelligence, tolerance of dysphoria, and coping skills serve them well. However, regardless of the healthiness of an individual's personality, no one is fully protected from the impact of severe forms of depression on functioning.

TABLE 4.2. Characteristics of "More Healthy" and "Less Healthy" Personalities

Relatively healthy/adaptive	Relatively unhealthy/maladaptive
Identity	
Sense of integrity	Diffuse sense of self
Strong beliefs	Unintegrated beliefs
Positive self-esteem	Sense of inadequacy,
Security and optimism about self	unlovability
and world	Insecurity and pessimism
Recognition and tolerance of	about self and world
vulnerability in self and	Emptiness, lack of self-
others	soothing
Self-nurturing	Need for "mirroring" to
Comfort with solitude	define self
Pleasure	No pleasure
Interpersonal skills	
Assertiveness	Passivity
Good communication	Poor communication skills
skills	Excessive sense of
Ability to give and take,	entitlement
share, cooperate	Jealousy, sensitivity to
Autonomy	rejection
Flexibility	Dependence, desperation
Enjoyment of intimacy/sex	Rigidity
Tolerance of conflict	Sexual conflict/blockage
Ability to trust	Intolerance of conflict
Gregariousness	Inability to trust
	Anxiety and avoidance
	Hostility, criticism
Productivity	
Creativity and curiosity	Lack of creativity, curiosity
Full use of potential	Blocked potential
Pleasure and satisfaction	No pleasure/satisfaction
in work	in work
Ability to play	Absence of playfulness
Perseverance and	Tendency to give up or
determination	become easily overwhelmed
Practicality	Limited practical capablities
Intelligence	Cognitive impairment
Energy	Listlessness, apathy
Decisiveness	Obsessionality
Coping skills (defenses)	
Humor	"Immature" or "primitive"
Altruism, mutuality	defenses
Sublimation, suppression	Acting out
Large capacity to tolerate and	Limited capacity to
modulate powerful affects	tolerate and modulate
	powerful affects

In our work in a medical school, we see many medical students and residents who are laboring under rather severe depressions. Most of them are able to maintain good levels of functioning at first, despite marked sleep disorder, anergy, and anhedonia, and various struggles with "existential" issues in their relationships and careers; they do not seek treatment until they begin to experience significant formal cognitive dysfunction. It is only then that they become overwhelmed in the face of weekly examinations with enormous amounts of new material to read and master, or the stress of making crucial life-saving decisions in the face of self-doubt and compromised thinking.

Healthy patients with depression often present a dilemma for clinicians, who find themselves talking with people who may be describing horrible symptoms but displaying minimal signs of depression. They come to evaluation and treatment with the same needs to stay "in control," to contain their vulnerability, to protect the therapist from empathic discomfort, and to avoid stigma as they demonstrate in other areas of their lives.

Depression in "Less Healthy" Personalities

Superimposing depression upon a relatively "unhealthy" personality structure results in a far more complex series of phenomena, with obviously more severe clinical ramifications. To start with, such people may already display (at least transiently or episodically) many of the manifestations of compromised interpersonal, identity-related, and work-related functions that are typical of depression. In fact, it is quite possible that many people with such characteristics have a chronic, low-grade primary mood disorder; these features may be either consequences of the continuing influence of the mood disturbance or early developmental adaptations to it.

Furthermore, an unhealthy personality by definition utilizes less mature defenses, has less margin for tolerance of affective changes, and is more likely to decompensate with less of an insult. As a result, the appearance of even the mildest symptoms of depression often results in significant compromise in each of the major areas of personality functioning. This may occur even in individuals with transient mood disturbances that are not reflective of the autonomous processes of illness. When more severe levels of depression occur in such people, there is usually severe regression: major disruption of or turmoil within relationships, total disability at work, and suicidal crises or perhaps even completed suicides. These are the people at the greatest risk from this illness.

Patients whose personality structures are on the less healthy side of the continuum often present a particular problem in assessment for clinicians. They may appear at a point of mild to moderate depression with clear and significant regression. In their assessment, they display profound neediness, manifested in hostile or clinging dependency, a sense of being overwhelmed, various forms of maladaptive acting out, productive paralysis, and/or suicidality. Since for most of us, the most powerful forces in shaping our convictions about people are our direct observations and experience, there is a common inclination to believe that "what you see is what you get." In this situation, the most provocative and powerful forces are often personality features, and these can lead the clinician mistakenly to identify a personality disorder to the exclusion of a mood disorder. That is, when patients present with a regressive picture driven by depression, it is tempting to look at the personality characteristics that are so visible and apparent and to assume that these represent the stable and usual configuration of personality structure. Clinicians who do not recognize state-dependent regressions of personality functions will be more likely to diagnose affectively disturbed patients as having borderline personality disorder. Underdiagnosis of depression is one consequence of this tendency. Another, alluded to above, involves the lack of suspicion of depression where the healthy personality is covering over and compensating for the disorder.

It is essential that clinicians always be vigilant for depression because of these masks and disguises. Particularly for a patient with clear personality problems, it becomes crucial to obtain a detailed history of state-dependent changes in personality functioning. Such historical information from the patient may be compromised by retroactive distortions created by the current depression, so that significant others may be necessary to help define the patient's "usual self." Many of these questions will be clarified during symptomatic remissions, as therapists working with depressed patients over time will experience them in both normal and regressed periods.

·5·

How to Conduct Biologically Informed Psychotherapy for Depression

GENERAL CONSIDERATIONS AND STRATEGIES

The conduct of biologically informed psychotherapy for depression (hereafter abbreviated as BIPD) involves the logical and systematic application of elements of several already existing methods of psychotherapy to patients whose depressive illnesses pervade their existence. Elements of psychodynamic therapy, cognitive-behavioral therapy (CBT), and interpersonal psychotherapy (IPT) are integrated with a continual orientation toward the biological nature of this final common pathway. It is this orientation toward the patient's biological depression as the central problem that helps guide the clinician throughout all phases of treatment.

In the course of studying and treating clinical depressive disorders over the past two decades, we have come to appreciate how much more recurrent and chronic these disorders are than they were originally believed to be. Patients with single episodes of depression are more the exception than the rule (Keller et al., 1984). As a consequence of this evolution in views, it behooves the clinician treating patients with depression to anticipate and prepare them for the likelihood that their illness may influence or punctuate their lives over both their immediate and long-term futures. This will rarely be news to such patients, as we frequently see people who have already been affected by their depressions for extended periods before seeking treatment or have already been in treatment on numerous occasions. Furthermore, the net of primary mood disorders has been spread wider, to incorporate both the milder forms of depression (Akiskal, 1983) and those problems that were formerly considered to be primarily personality disorders but in which regressive experiences are fueled by depression. For example, before 1980 and the introduction of DSM-III, what we now call dysthymic disorder was considered either a nervous or a characterological problem. Similarly, before DSM-IV placed it in an appendix for further study, minor depressive disorder had no place in the official nosology.) The fact of having a depressive episode implies a vulnerability to depression that will not disappear. Although there are suggestions that early medical and psychotherapeutic interventions may diminish the likelihood of recurrence, there are no absolute preventative measures. Therefore, rational strategies for treating depression must include both short-term and long-term planning.

Considerations for the use of antidepressant medications have reflected rational and other processes operating within both therapists and patients. The efficacy of antidepressants in the treatment of depression is unquestionable (American Psychiatric Association, 1993). In studies comparing the use of antidepressants with both CBT and IPT, all three treatments have been shown to be quite effective in treating milder forms of depression (Elkin et al., 1989); antidepressant medications show greater efficacy than either CBT or IPT in more severe forms of major depression. Some studies (Frank et al., 1990; Kupfer et al., 1992) have demonstrated a distinct advantage of combining psychotherapies with medications in both resolving acute episodes of depression and preventing recurrence. Although the BIPD approach incorporates the use of medications into psychotherapy, we recognize that an antidepressant medication may not be an active component in treatment at various stages of remission or at times when only the milder forms of depression are present. However, even when antidepressants are not actively in use, they should always be "under consideration," and this "consideration" as well as their active use is central to treatment strategies. Practically, these medications work to control symptoms and prevent recurrences. Theoretically, they reverse the pathological processes that underlie depression.

Given a disorder that has a tendency toward chronicity and recurrence, and whose consequences are potentially so far-reaching and profound, the overall strategy of treatment involves developing a partnership between therapist and patient in which their mutual goals are as follows:

1. To understand depression and its idiosyncratic impact on this patient.
2. To control its acute symptoms and to limit relapse and recurrence.
3. To minimize its consequences for the patient in the world ("damage control").

The elements of BIPD are derived from the implementation of this overall strategy. These elements are nothing more than systematic, practical techniques designed to correct the problems created by depression. Because the quality, time course, and consequences of depression are so variable, the application of these treatment methods will vary from individual to individual. The specific techniques used at any point in time depend upon the course of the patient's illness, the effectiveness of communication between therapist and patient, and the patient's and therapist's abilities to solve problems. The adoption of an integrated biopsychosocial perspective should facilitate this process for both therapist and patient.

Central to any discussion of treatment strategies is the development of a strong working relationship between patient and therapist. The psychotherapist must have qualities that will help him or her develop, maintain, and sustain a relationship in which the other person is at times suffering greatly, usually seeking support and remediation. These qualities include empathy; understanding of depression; patience and perseverance; a strong desire to help; and the skills to explore, confront, contradict, and at times cajole. A good working alliance requires a concurrence of purposes and goals between patient and therapist. This can only be achieved through the patient's comfort with and trust and confidence in the therapist, as well as the therapist's active education of the patient about the nature of this treatment.

The psychotherapeutic components of the BIPD approach address the goals outlined above in repetitive, overlapping, and reinforcing ways, which we describe in this chapter. Interwoven with all of these strategies is psychopharmacological treatment, especially for moderate and severe levels of depression (and frequently for milder forms). The strategies are as follows:

1. Education
2. Psychodynamic exploration
3. Coping skills exploration, training, and support
4. Work with significant others
5. Psychotherapy in connection with psychopharmacological treatment
6. Management of suicidality

EDUCATION

The role of education in the psychotherapy of depression is paramount. It is a continual process that informs both patient and therapist about the nature of the patient's depression; the forces that precipitate, maintain, or aggravate the disorder; both patients' efforts to change the patient's state of mind, self-perceptions, interactions, and role functions; and the patient's efforts to tolerate this state, distract himself or herself from it, or flee from it in various forms. In many ways, all of the psychotherapeutic approaches discussed in this chapter entail elements of education.

Teaching can be one of the tools for the therapist to engage the patient and begin to enhance the therapeutic alliance in the earliest phases of assessment. When a patient begins to discuss aspects of his or her depression, the knowledgeable and skilled therapist will use an understanding of the disorder to inquire about the details of depression in a way that will enrich the clinical material being presented, as well as increase the patient's appreciation of the therapist's understanding of his or her state of mind. Most clinicians begin their assessments with open-ended inquiries about the nature of their patients' problems, and are told about some combinations of circumstances and symptoms that are troubling and often confusing. When clinical depression is part of the picture, this may be experienced by the patients as overwhelming or out of their control—which is often the case. Following such a patient's initial presentation, a clinician has an opportunity, through systematic inquiry into the symptoms and "language" of depression, to bring some greater degree of organization to the myriad of disconnected complaints. The patient's endorsement of symptoms and depression-related problems is helpful in a number of ways. It is reassuring to know that the clinician appreciates what is wrong. The patient can further infer from this inquiry that there is a general body of knowledge somewhere about this condition. By communicating effectively during the interview, the therapist can begin to engage the patient in some of the more therapeutic ways of thinking about the depression and its impact on his or her life, particularly the central role of the depression itself. Examples of this type of inquiry can be seen in the following therapist comments and questions:

"You're describing a lot of depression. How has it affected your marriage?"
"When people are depressed, they can become irritable or short-tempered. Have these problems happened to you with other people?"
"Since you've been depressed, you say that you've lost your sense of humor. Have you also found every interaction to be a hassle? . . . Become more clingy than usual?"

These are fairly general questions that both identify the depression and introduce it as a possible causal agent in other areas of difficulty.

Depending on the person's ability to respond or the type of response, the therapist may become more detailed or pointed in the inquiry. These questions also communicate to the patient that depression is an entity; that it acts upon people and can change the ways they feel and behave; and that there is something "normative" about the patient's behavior, even if it isn't "normal" for him or her. The matter-of-factness about, empathy for, and acceptance of these phenomena conveyed in the therapist's communications will help the patient to modify his or her experience. Through a systematic inquiry into the symptoms and language of depression, the assessment phase not only can be deepened and enriched, but can itself prove to be therapeutic to the patient, can strengthen the therapeutic alliance, and can increase the patient's motivation for further treatment.

Symptoms

Education that focuses on the recognition of the symptoms of depression serves numerous functions. Most importantly, symptoms are the current means of diagnosing a depressive disorder. Once a patient has experienced depression and it goes into remission, the reappearance of these symptoms can suggest the ineffectiveness of the current treatment or, in the absence of treatment, the spontaneous recurrence of the disorder. Furthermore, the level of depression can be monitored through the presence or intensity of various symptoms. Patients tend to have similar patterns in the sequence of symptom recruitment from one episode to the next, often reflecting the depth of their depression. These patterns and their intensity help to guide a patient and therapist in decisions about the frequency and types of therapy, institution of or change in use of psychopharmacological agents, and environmental changes that are likely to be beneficial to the patient.

It seems self-evident that patients can learn to recognize and monitor these symptoms as a means of achieving knowledge and mastery. However, unless this is done in a systematic and almost disciplined way, and often even when it is done in this way, the patient remains at risk of becoming a "captive" of the depression. The power of the emotional and physical state overcomes the patient's capacity to reflect upon what is happening, undermines his or her ability or willingness to communicate this to the therapist, or leaves the patient apathetic or hopeless about being able to make any changes, thereby disrupting the treatment that can help him or her.

For these reasons, regular and systematic review of symptoms should be incorporated into standard procedures as a component of treatment and monitoring. One method of increasing the patient's ability and willingness to watch for and recognize symptom patterns (beyond time in the office) can be the regular use of standardized self-report symptom checklists, such as the Beck Depression Inventory (Beck et al., 1961) or the Zung Self-Rating Depression Scale (Zung, 1965). An alternative might be to develop a personalized inventory that emphasizes the clinical features of greatest significance to the patient. Although the primary purposes of such scrutiny are understanding, monitoring, and maintaining perspective, an additional benefit is the utilization of obsessional mechanisms to bind the painful affects of depression and to create a productive activity.

Scientific Education

Once the diagnosis of a clinical depression (whether major depressive disorder, the depressed phase of a bipolar illness, or dysthymic disorder) has been established, some formal education about depression is in order. This can proceed in a number of different ways, depending upon the inclinations and abilities of the patient. The patient has a condition about which a great deal is known in terms of its incidence, prevalence, manifestations, and course with various treatments. Much is also known about what its nature is and is not. Depending on the clinician's knowledge, comfort, and skills at informing patients about depression, it is useful to develop a brief talk that can be given to patients (and their families when this is indicated). Although there are numerous theoretical models for understanding the biology of depression (see Chapter 1), the catecholamine hypothesis is the most popular and can be explained as the "best guess," with the aid of diagrams such as Figure 1.1 or the use of fingers to simulate a synapse and explain in a simplified way how a neurotransmitter functions. It is very helpful to have a bibliography to refer to or to give directly to patients, listing books on depression at various levels of sophistication and with various technical/scientific, phenomenological, or biographical orientations. Patients should be encouraged to learn as much as they can about their disorder, so that they can develop as much of a collaborative relationship as possible with their therapists. Although patients may not have therapists' expertise and do need therapists' independent judgment and feedback, such participation will enhance their motivation for and compliance with treatment, encourage a sense of greater autonomy and mastery, and diminish the degree of unnecessary dependency on the therapists. Most important, this formal education enhances the patients' understanding of a disorder with which they must familiarize themselves in order to limit its impact on their lives.

One of the educational functions of therapists is to dispel patients' almost inevitable misconceptions about their disorder. We have chosen to approach this proactively and aggressively, recognizing that our patients often perceive their depressions as manifestations of moral failure and personal weakness or inadequacy; they feel that they have brought this on themselves or that they deserve their suffering. The advantages of anticipating these beliefs are (1) that it serves to normalize them and (2) that although it does not invalidate the experience of these beliefs, it contributes to an earlier start to undermining them and replacing them with more valid and helpful views.

A view about depression held by many patients and some therapists is that it is produced by some deep-seated conflict or issue, which can only be cured by the equivalent of psychological exorcism. Discouraged by the suffering they have encountered, skeptical of a process that they only vaguely understand and that is often a subject of derision, and pessimistic about their own capacity to change, patients may approach treatment with great reservations. Redefining the nature of the disorder and describing the effectiveness of pharmacological and psychological therapies can often bring hope to the hopeless.

Translating and Reinterpreting the Language of Depression

An essential element of patient education involves learning the "language" of depression, for the purposes of translating and reinterpreting it in ways that will be most adaptive and least disruptive to a patient's life. In Chapter 4, we have examined the numerous and varied ways in which depression manifests itself in changes in the depressed patient's identity and world view, relationships, and productive activities. It is clear that depression can insinuate itself into and undermine any area of living, including life itself. Depression can create a variety of illusions in any of these spheres, which, if acted upon, can lead to enormous damage to a patient's work, relationships, and self. It is bad enough that the depressed person feels terrible, but worse still that the depression can ruin his or her life. Translating and reinterpreting the language of depression can thus serve major functions in "damage control."

The process of learning the language of depression begins at the first evaluation sessions and remains a continuing focus throughout treatment. Every session involves some review of the patient's areas of functioning; the patient and therapist look in detail at how elements of depression express themselves in both subtle and obvious ways. For this kind of exploration, a therapist should have familiarity with this language in order to direct it. As time goes on, the patient can take more responsibility for this examination. However, the limiting factor for the patient is always likely to be the loss of perspective created by the depression, as the following two examples demonstrate.

> For many years, Ted's depression was heralded by a "black cloud" of irritability, which was quickly focused on his wife. He would seethe and, with or without provocation, inevitably have an explosion. His experience while depressed was one of justified resentment. When the depression passed, he invariably felt humiliated and realized that his explosion had been unwarranted. However, the marital relationship suffered from the immediate and residual effects of his explosions. Treatment with antidepressants diminished the frequency and intensity of his depression. Of greater importance to him was the ability to identify depression at the moment and find alternate means of dealing with his resentment. He still felt the resentment and *felt* it was justified, but was able to carry on an internal argument about whether it was legitimate, with increasing awareness that his anger was an artifact—a by-product of his depression.

> Phillip is now a professional in his late 30s whose recurrent depression formerly stifled his relationships, career, and self-esteem. (His case is described in greater detail in Chapter 8.) During periods of marked depression, he experienced a profound paralysis and impaired concentration, accompanied by self-deprecation, doubts about his career path, and perceptions of failure. At such times he would stop working, all forces of depression conspiring to undermine any reasons to work. Despite considerable treatment, with dramatic positive changes in his self-concept, relationships, and work, there are still periods when depression asserts itself and leaves him feeling depleted. However, his response now is this: "It's the depression again; it seems to make work almost impossible." He does his work against this gradient, aware that the way he feels has no particular meaning beyond the primary experience. He knows he can do the work and has a sense of accomplishment for his efforts.

These two vignettes have been selected to demonstrate a central feature of treatment: Perspective is crucial to functioning. Patients with depression must learn to identify the many manifestations of their disorder and to reinterpret the phenomena in terms of their more fundamental meaning: "It's the depression talking!" This is an essential translation for patients to learn, both as a means of identifying the depression for purposes of treating it, and as a means of undermining the apparent "moral imperative" of a state of mind that threatens relationships, work, and life. The following examples further emphasize the issues driven by patients' depressions and presenting as existential dilemmas demanding immediate, far-reaching, and potentially destructive solutions.

Robin and Jeff had a stable, caring marriage, which was punctuated by Robin's episodes of depression. During these periods, she saw Jeff's quiet, reserved nature as deliberately withholding; his usual independence as a lack of intimacy; and his usually mildly annoying habits as personal assaults. She pressed for divorce.

Ed was a medical resident who had recently moved from another city, where he'd had an excellent record in medical school, good friends, and enthusiasm about his future. After several weeks of frequent on-call duty and other highly demanding responsibilities, he developed a sleep and appetite disturbance; became increasingly depressed, anergic, and anhedonic; and finally became cognitively impaired. Although he realized he was depressed, he was certain he should drop out of his training and enter a nonmedical field. Why? Because he was incapable of being a doctor; he was afraid of making the wrong decisions; he wasn't sure that he hadn't gone to medical school just to please his parents.

The therapist's dilemma in cases such as Robin's and Ed's usually focuses on at least one of two issues. First, without a clear recognition of the role of depression in shaping such patients' perceptions of these problems, the therapist may not even be aware that depression exists. Under such circumstances, it is common for the clinician to focus on the merits of the existential dilemma (in these two cases, whether to stay married, whether to leave medicine) and develop treatment designed to answer such questions. Even when patients do not recognize the elements of depression and relate material to the therapist that is solely focused on the apparent existential issues, it is essential for the clinician to maintain a strong index of suspicion of the possibility of depression and to pursue its inquiry vigorously.

Once there is a clear recognition of how powerfully these patients' "decisions" are being forced by the depression itself, the immediate clinical intervention involves the identification of these driving forces and *active* dismissal of the need to answer the questions immediately. The issues should be deferred until the depression is treated, since there is a good chance that the patients' "dilemmas" will dissolve when their depression subsides. This leads to the therapist's other dilemma.

Traditionally, psychotherapists have been trained to be patient observers and good, empathic listeners. They are expected to be emotionally supportive, accepting, inquiring, and (occasionally) confronting and interpreting. A premium has been placed on patients' self-direction, self-inquiry, and autonomy in decision making. The approach we are advocating here in treating depressed patients demands that in addition to having these necessary qualities, therapists challenge patients' perceptions of many of their problems and confront them with the possibility or likelihood that they are seeing things incorrectly. This may be perceived as therapists' intruding with their expertise and judgments, being parental, and/or exerting efforts to control and change their patients' perceptions. They may appear to be infantilizing their adult patients in ways that do not come easily to people in the mental health field. Such approaches are antithetical to the personal and treatment philosophies of many therapists.

How can this dilemma be resolved? The answer to this emanates from our conceptualization of overall strategy. Depression is the enemy. It is an entity that imposes itself on people and distorts their being. The task for therapists is to develop a treatment alliance with their patients in order to control the depression, to understand and quiet or undermine its voice, and to limit its impact on the victims. This requires constant vigilance on the therapists' part to identify the manifestations of depression and confront their effects. This can become an educational project for both therapists and patients. As patients reorient themselves to such issues, they come to recognize and accept that such confrontations by their therapists, or ultimately by themselves, do not undermine their autonomy or diminish them as people. Instead, there is a growing awareness that they are not defined by these depressive perceptions. Initially through their therapists' eyes, and later through their own, they are able to see that they have a *core self*, an undepressed self, that is quite different from the depressed self. Over time, the distorted language of depression becomes more ego-dystonic, and confrontations are seen as directed to the depressed self. The following are hypothetical therapist replies to the dilemmas of Robin and Ed, above. Each one demonstrates both the recognition of depression's role in the dilemma and an argument against acting upon it, while underscoring that the therapist's argument is not with the person but with the effects of the depression.

THERAPIST: Robin, I've known you for a while, and I've seen you go through the same sequence of events on a number of occasions. I know you and Jeff have difficulties, but they seem to get blown way out of proportion when your depression worsens. I think it would be a mistake to act on these feelings right now. Once your mood is better, you may feel differently. That will be a better time to decide whether your marriage is or is not in your long-term interest.

THERAPIST: Ed, since we've never met before, I can't appreciate whether or not it makes sense for you to leave medicine now. I do know that for most people who have gotten this far, it requires a lot of ability, determination, and motivation, so I can't imagine that you've arrived here without a lot of good reasons. On the other hand, I've seen what depression can do to undermine a person's work [the therapist gives details], motivation [details], and confidence [details]. Rather than make any long-term decision, let's see if you can get some leave time, treat the depression aggressively, and then see how you feel when you're not in the throes of such an awful state.

In each of these responses, the therapist takes a conservative stance about the patient's dilemma: "Don't act until you are no longer depressed." It is done with the understanding that there is pathology at work pressing for a decision that may be harmful, and with the assumption that the patient's perceptions will change in a different state of mind. It is a response similar to the advice of a wise grandparent, hearing of middle-of-the-night turmoil: "Wait to see how you feel in the morning."

Another important technical element in each of these replies is the therapist's allying himself or herself with the patient's strengths, obtained in the first instance through direct observation and in the second through inference. This becomes a way of underscoring the therapist's genuine belief in the patient's "core" abilities (as opposed to his or her "depression-compromised" abilities). It requires that the therapist be able to sort through all of the patient's "depression-compromised" qualities and see such strengths. Certainly this is a universal requirement of all forms of psychotherapy. It is also attainable, since there is good in all people and strength in all people. The impediments to such perceptions are usually reflections of problems within the therapist.

As a therapist and patient work together over time on translating the language of depression and attempting to correct its distortions, the capacity of the therapist to provide this "undistorted mirror" function is crucial. With time and greater depth of knowledge and understanding about the patient, the therapist will have an increasing conviction about the patient's "core," and may have to use this conviction to combat the effects of depression. At times the depression will even distort the patient's efforts at interpreting its effects. For example:

PATIENT: I'm convinced that I really can't proceed. I just don't have the ability.

THERAPIST: I think that's a reflection of your mood. Last month you were feeling better and you were getting work done, feeling optimistic. Nothing is different now except your mood.

PATIENT: Well, maybe last month was the illusion and this month is the truth.

What is the therapist to do? On the one hand, it is clear that the patient's concluding remark continues to reflect depression, but might it also reflect some truth? Therapists may experience this quandary and be paralyzed by indecision because of their inability to define an absolute truth that will help such patients. We all appreciate the contradictory and ambivalent in ourselves, our relationships, our principles, and our institutions.

In our work of translating the effects of depression, we find that the better replies are those that lead patients to the most adaptive stances or perceptions. Such a reply can and should acknowledge both elements of a patient's perceptions, but emphasize what will be "healthier." Many types of therapist responses might reflect this:

> "Sure, many things are possible, but your life seemed a lot better for you last month. I'm voting for that illusion."
> "Regardless of how you see things now, I still see someone who has the capacity to do what you set out to do."
> "Well, you may see yourself going down the toilet right now, and maybe a lot of life is shitty, but I'll bet we will have a very different conversation about this in the near future."

Each of these responses confronts the distortions created by the depression, presents the therapist's convictions about the patient's strengths, and offers hope. The specific content of such responses is shaped by the material presented, the nature of the therapeutic relationship, aspects of the therapist's personality and style, the patient's sensitivities, and more. The message to be conveyed must be heard, and the therapist's creativity and skill at being heard are crucial.

Because of the centrality and constancy of the therapist's perception about the patient's "core," the person of the therapist also takes on a more substantial reality in BIPD than in other forms of psychotherapy. The therapist's views are important and indeed often necessary; as such, they are introduced with great regularity until they can be incorporated by the patient. Although these views are presented in more explicit ways than in traditional psychodynamic therapies, they play a role similar to the therapist's role in such treatments, where the therapist may be incorporated and later integrated as an "internal object representation" or in a "mirroring transference" that becomes a stable part of the self (see, e.g., Kohut, 1971, 1977). The stability and constancy of the therapist's perceptions in BIPD convey his or her respect and appreciation for the patient's positive capacities. They also counterbalance the confronting, challenging, and more parental functions that are inherent elements of interpreting the language of depression.

Let us consider briefly the consequences of a therapist's adopting a more traditional stance with a patient who is quite depressed and making a mood-driven decision. The patient's decision is quite consistent with the perceptions that are being presented. A dynamically oriented, biologically uninformed therapist may perceive, as does the patient, that the depression is a consequence of a conflictual situation from which the patient should extricate himself or herself. Although the therapist may have some reservations about the patient's decision, the therapist is likely not only to avoid interjecting his or her own belief system, but, acting on the (usually) laudable principles that "patients know their needs best" and "autonomy is paramount," to support or endorse the patient's decision. However, mood-driven decisions are made by depressed patients because they hope that what is making them unhappy will change as a result of the decision, or because the dysfunction created by the depression has forced them into such a position. Although occasionally such decisions turn out fine, the usual consequences of these are the losses of jobs, relationships, or family and other supports. These often lead to greater instability, to worsening symptoms or more regressive adaptations, and to further mood-driven decisions (up to and including suicide).

It is essential that clinicians working with the depressed appreciate the serious consequences of their own passivity and indecision. Errors of omission in the name of respect for patients' autonomy are common. Depressed patients require therapists who are active allies—advocates against a disorder that truly robs them of their autonomy. Therapists must be willing to confront, challenge, and "fight" with patients to help them see the impact of depression on all aspects of their lives, and to combat it aggressively (including medically).

PSYCHODYNAMIC EXPLORATION

Although the view of psychodynamic exploration as the sole means of understanding and "working through" the "causes" of depression in order to "cure" a patient is no longer a tenable stance, there remain important applications of psychodynamic principles within an integrated psychotherapeutic approach to this disorder.

As we have emphasized throughout this book, many factors contribute to depressive illness. These include genetic and developmental vulnerabilities and insults; hormonal and other internal biological alterations; and precipitating events. The predisposing factors of genetics and development may be amenable to exploration and some level of understanding, but are unchangeable in their fundamental existence. A patient's genetic contribution may be alterable in the future, but it is fixed now; a parental death will not "unhappen." There are, however, numerous ways in which developmental issues and maladaptively resolved conflicts can intrude into the present and play a role in the shaping of psychopathology, even though such forces do not cause the illness. Dynamic forces can influence a person's response to depression, the content of his or her depressive language, and the efforts to treat them. An understanding of psychodynamics can be applied to many different aspects of depression and its treatment:

1. Psychodynamic issues as stressors
2. Universal and idiosyncratic dynamics of responses to illness
3. Interpreting the language of regression
4. "Historical revisionism" (i.e., exploration of depression's impact on development)
5. Psychodynamics of psychopharmacological treatment
6. Psychodynamics of the patient–therapist relationship

Psychodynamic Issues as Stressors

Traditional views of psychopathology have depicted depression as a direct manifestation of psychodynamic conflict. Through loss or deprivation (Freud 1917/1957), impaired self-esteem (Bibring, 1953), retroflexed anger (Abraham, 1911/1948), and other mechanisms, unconscious anxiety has been thought to be transformed into a particular disorder—in this case, depression. Because of the centrality of these forces in the development of pathology in traditional psychodynamic approaches, most of the treatment effort in these approaches is directed at uncovering and "working through" these issues. Other efforts and interventions, such as "support," advice, education, and psychopharmacology, are seen as distractions from the primary process. These distractions are thought to provide only "palliation" and transient benefits (as opposed to the presumed "curative" nature of analytically oriented treatment). Most importantly, they are felt to interfere with the treatment by changing the nature of the transference and altering the transference neurosis, which is viewed as the vehicle for cure (Rounsaville et al., 1981).

The changing role of dynamic exploration in treating depression is a direct reflection of changing views of the psychopathology of this disorder. Dynamic forces have come to be seen less as idiosyncratic and symbolic contributions to the development of depression than as nonspecific stressors with cumulative power. Developmental issues of loss, distrust, entitlement, impaired self-esteem, conflicts with authority, heightened dependency, and so forth are played out in daily living in ways that are directly maladaptive and that undermine stability and satisfaction with life. Such factors are inherently troublesome and upsetting to people and may warrant treatment. However, their effect on depression is at most indirect—the result of continuing stresses created by threatened or lost relationships, financial insecurity from loss of work, or the weight of ongoing disruption over time (Paykel et al., 1969; Kendler et al., 1993). In such circumstances, exploration of disruptive dynamic forces for the purpose of understanding and ultimately changing these maladaptive behaviors may lower the chances that depression will be expressed in vulnerable individuals, but cannot reverse a process that has become an autonomous one, even in cases where such forces are operating strongly.

How much time and effort goes into the exploration of these stressors should reflect the extent to which they are deemed to contribute to the depression. Several considerations influence this decision. Although many people suffering from depression appear to be sensitive to stress in the precipitation of or aggravation of depressive episodes, there are also a substantial number of people (particularly those with stronger genetic influences) whose depressions wax and wane on principles as yet unfathomable, seemingly driven by some internal mechanisms. Others seem influenced by more clear-cut biological variables, such as seasonal changes in exposure to sunlight, or changes related to hormonal variations associated with menses, childbirth, or menopause in many women. Moreover, once a depressive diathesis has developed, repeated episodes of depression and a future chronic course are likely to evolve with much less "push" from the environment (Post et al., 1981).

For other patients, depression-precipitating psychosocial stressors may be either unpredictable, uncontrollable, catastrophic forces or the mundane and inherent stresses of normal daily living. With either of these kinds of stressors, extensive dynamic exploration for the purpose of reducing risks would seem to be of limited value. All experienced psychotherapists understand the tenacity of maladaptive behaviors, their resistance to change, and the enormous effort necessary to accomplish such change. Clearly, if a therapist assumes that such changes are essential and central to the treatment of depression, the devastating nature of the disorder justifies such effort. However, if a therapist's estimate of the influence of such forces in producing the disorder is reduced from the figure of perhaps 80–100% to one of only 0–20%, estimates of the amount of effort that needs to be invested in changing these forces for risk management purposes may decrease proportionately. The actual determination of the contribution of such factors to risk is not easy or exact, but should be based on strong historical correlations with exacerbations of symptoms—not on tautological reasoning, as has so often been the case. Kendler et al. (1992) found that among a group of approximately 1,000 women who were monozygotic or dizygotic twins, the contribution of the death or divorce of a parent before age 18, though statistically significant in the development of a subsequent depressive episode, had only 4% of the impact of genetic factors in the development of depression.

From a practical standpoint, the examination of both mundane and extraordinary current life stressors can serve many purposes. Most obviously, a review of those forces that are having a significant ongoing psychological impact on the patient can help the therapist and patient deepen their understanding of the patient's mental life. This appreciation can be of heuristic value; more importantly, it can expand the bases for knowledge about the patient's state-dependent experiences, whether the state is one of depression or normality. In either case, this is useful information for the present and future.

Following current events and the patient's reactions to them can also be another means of monitoring the patient's progress in treating and coping with the depression. Furthermore, for those patients who are in the throes of moderate to severe depression and whose perspective and coping skills have been compromised, explorations and discussions of such stressors may be necessary to promote continued functioning or to prevent deterioration. Finally, some stressors, as determined by historical data, can actually precipitate or exacerbate symptoms of depression. The identification of these, and adaptive interventions for them, may have protective value for the patient.

There also are reasons why, beyond identification, the exploration of and intervention with stressors may be harmful. For example, when a relatively "healthy" (see Chapter 4) patient is in remission from depression and functioning at full capacity, we are disinclined to spend much time or effort looking at "depression-unrelated" problems at work or home. Instead, we convey that this is an area that the patient is quite capable of attending to alone, without the help of a mental health professional. We feel that this is supportive of the patient's health and autonomy—areas that have been under sufficient assault by the depressive illness. This active and selective use of "benign neglect" should be openly conveyed to reinforce its purpose.

Universal and Idiosyncratic Dynamics of Responses to Illness

Helping depressed patients to integrate an understanding of the dynamics of their responses to depression into their identity and world view is a recurring theme in treatment. Many responses to the existence of a depressive illness (in contrast to the more direct effects of the illness), or to almost any recurrent or chronic and potentially debilitating illness, are universal, predictable, and normal. Others are unique to the individuals involved.

People with chronic illness will normally experience some impairment or compromise in self-esteem—a narcissistic injury to the always perpetuated illusion of invulnerability. This is the kind of defect or disability that is easier to hide than a clubfoot or cerebral palsy, and it is the usual response of people with depression to hide their disorder from others (including, at times, those who could help them). The urge to hide is clearly reinforced by social stigma and at times even by therapists, as they may be reluctant to "hurt" their patients by rubbing the patients' noses in their "defect." On the other hand, the control of depression and prevention of morbidity and mortality in this disorder do not permit our denial of this continuing vulnerability as a defect. Part of successful treatment does involve helping depressed patients accept the reality that they have a chronic illness. Ironically, though also logically, the acceptance of the disorder can lead to the minimization of its negative impact through effective treatment.

In regard to this particular issue, life may be much more comfortable when both therapist and patient are able to share the myth of personal control conferred by the notion that "where id was, there let ego be." Despite the degree of suffering, there is the conviction or hope that sufficiently thorough understanding will "cure" the problem. When depression remits, either spontaneously or in relation to the treatment, patients are spared the confrontation with their fixed vulnerability until the next episode. Those in whom depression persists, however, may be further injured by the sense of their own failure to accept or be effective (i.e., their "resistance") in the analytically oriented treatment—views that are reinforced by central tenets of analytically oriented treatment.

As a young rabbinical student, Alan had experienced a devastating depression that left him seriously impaired in his studies and persistently contemplating suicide. He entered twice-weekly exploratory psychotherapy over the next 2 years, without psychopharmacological intervention. His depression persisted throughout the first year of treatment, during 9 months of which his suicidal preoccupation continued. When he finally completed his treatment, he was highly appreciative of the help and understanding he had received from his therapist. But an exacerbation of depression a few years later left him feeling perplexed, helpless, and betrayed. How had this happened? Hadn't he "worked through" the issues within himself and with his family sufficiently? Did he need more work? Alan's second depressive episode responded quickly and fully to antidepressant treatment, leaving him fully functional and feeling good about himself and his life. However, he now perceived himself vulnerable in a way that was disconcerting: He had an illness that was difficult for him to accept. He had been much more reassured, prior to its exacerbation, that he had simply had problems that could be overcome with patience, the hard work of exploration, and his faith. It is in the nature of depression to deceive patient and therapist alike. Spontaneous remissions seem to confirm the value of any concurrent activity.

Interacting with this universal dynamic of impaired self-esteem are individual, idiosyncratic dynamic themes. Those patients with more blatant narcissistic disorders are likely to have a more difficult time accepting the fact of their depression and may seek refuge in other, "kinder" explanations. Those with more obsessional and controlling qualities may also fight more strongly against the concept of an illness that is beyond their personal control, especially the notion that medication may be necessary for their well-being. This is especially ironic, in light of the reality that the basic objective of scientific medicine is to bring understanding and control where disease reigns. Over time, obsessional patients do tend to gravitate toward this view, especially when they find treatments that are effective.

It should be noted that when we talk about dynamic factors in more "narcissistic" and "obsessional" patients, we are identifying people who exhibit a greater resistance to seeing their depression as an illness, rather than people whose depression is a direct consequence of their personality structure. This latter traditional view is not supported by data: Character structure does not cause depression. Such people's personality structures may explain why, in the face of disappointment, failure, rejection or other out-of-control events, they tend to get upset: They have farther to fall, because of the demandingness and inflexibility of their ego ideals. However, being upset is not the same as being clinically depressed.

Operating simultaneously with heightened vulnerability is the dependency that is normally triggered by illness (as well as dysfunction). Those patients with the strongest baseline characteristics of dependency will feel more comfortable with this state than more counterdependent types (obsessional and narcissistic), and are more likely to seek out and comply with treatment.

Interpreting the Language of Regression

Another important type of psychodynamic exploration, within the broader process of education, is the examination by therapist and patient of the developmental levels of a patient's achievement throughout the spectrum of psychodynamic issues. In practice, treatment examines the most primitive and regressive manifestations up through the most mature manifestations of the patient's conflicts: from inadequacy and dependency to autonomy and self-reliance; from undifferentiation to identity differentiation to integration; from insecurity to trust to intimacy; and so on. The Eriksonian model of identity formation (Erikson, 1950) can serve as a structure for this therapeutic task (see Table 5.1). The task is to identify not only those regressive positions that are manifestations of depression, but the highest developmental levels that represent the patient's healthy accomplishments. The purpose of this endeavor is ultimately for the therapist and patient to be able to use such information as a weapon in their efforts to counter the forces of depression as it speaks in yet another language. Depression's treachery is compounded by the reality that whatever form of regression is manifested, it has a reality base in development that resonates with the destructive distortions produced by the depression, as the next two examples demonstrate.

Joan had overcome childhood deprivation and abuse, had raised two children, and had worked effectively for many years. She had one failed marriage, but a subsequent successful relationship of long standing. Her self-image was largely positive. However, exacerbations of depression triggered old and familiar experiences of being inadequate, overwhelmed, unlovable, and intensely dependent. These feelings dovetailed with her anergy and anhedonia to push her toward withdrawal from her loved ones and work. From repeated experience, Joan and her therapist were able to recognize that these regressive states did not reflect her true self. She was able to fight against such inclinations and

TABLE 5.1. The Language of Regression: Effects of Depressive Regressions on Eriksonian Developmental Stages

Eriksonian developmental stage	Successful resolution	Regressive outcome
I. Trust versus mistrust	Drive and hope	Anergy, apathy, and fear
II. Autonomy versus shame and doubt	Self-control and will-power	Dependency and helplessness
III. Initiative versus guilt	Direction and purpose	Paralysis, fear, and guilt
IV. Industry versus inferiority	Method and competence	Incompetence and inferiority
V. Identity versus role confusion	Devotion and fidelity	Disintegration and confusion
VI. Intimacy versus isolation	Affiliation and love	Isolation and unlovability
VII. Generativity versus stagnation	Production and care	Emptiness and apathy
VIII. Ego integrity versus despair	Renunciation and wisdom	Meaninglessness and despair

Note. The "eight stages of man" (I–VIII) are the universal developmental conflicts described by Erikson (1950). The successful outcomes are those suggested by Erikson and the regressive outcomes are those suggested by him and extended by the authors.

keep working, caring for her loved ones, and staying involved, despite how bad she felt.

Lorraine had overcome long-standing feelings of insecurity and inadequacy, and was working effectively as a school principal. Her work demanded that she be confident and assertive in confronting daily problems with students, teachers, and the school bureaucracy. When episodes of depression occurred, she would again experience feelings of inadequacy, would doubt her decisions, and would become convinced that she didn't belong in this important position. Her awareness, through treatment, of the state-dependent nature of these feelings and the time-tested reality of her competence allowed her to "act" competently even at those times when she wasn't feeling that way.

In each of these examples, there was yet another set of factors—beyond symptoms and dimensions of functioning—that was distorted by depression and required monitoring and correcting. The systematic exploration of developmental dynamic issues in cases such as these allows both therapist and patient to achieve a deeper and richer grasp of depressive phenomena and their nondepressed counterparts. This understanding does not lead to cure, but helps patients to understand and tolerate the state they are in—and, more importantly, to avoid acting upon their depression-driven distortions, which would create even more detrimental circumstances.

Historical Revisionism

"Historical revisionism" refers to the reexamination of a depressed person's development with an effort to understand depression's impact on development. This type of psychodynamic exploration is pursued with those people who have lived with depression throughout much of their lives, including their childhoods. This exploration focuses not on the dynamic "origins" of depression, but on those developmental issues and experiences that have been influenced by depression and that, in turn have shaped the patients' current lives. Through this approach to exploration, which emphasizes a biological perspective on depression and its impact, such patients often develop a very different view of themselves. It is usually a more empathic and forgiving view than the harsh, critical, self-deprecating, and self-blaming views of children with depression who become adults with depression.

This reexamination of a patient's life experiences often proceeds against the litany of a lifetime of misattribution. Pejorative views of "laziness," "nastiness," "inattentiveness," "social inadequacy," and "stupidity" are reexamined as manifestations of an illness. The patient can come to see himself or herself as a victim, not an offender. A general sense of failure can be reinterpreted in terms of valiant efforts to compensate for overwhelming circumstances. Anything the patient has accomplished has been achieved in the face of great adversity—a struggle against a steep gradient.

Given common genetic threads, such children may also have had parents suffering from depression, and this exploration may yield a more compassionate understanding of both the affected parents and the impact of having such parents on the children's own lives. Even "normal" parents have limited capacities in dealing with depressed children. Understanding this from an adult perspective may soften some of the grown-up children's residual pain.

It is important also to recognize that some of the consequences of childhood depression may be positive. For instance, the children may have learned to be more compassionate as people. In addition, depressed children may develop coping skills that contribute greatly to their abilities in adulthood to tolerate affect, to learn means of escape, and to make adaptive use of solitude.

A risk of historical revisionism, as well as of redefining patients' perceptions of their depression, is that the individuals will come to see themselves as "flawed" in some unchangeable way and will "give in" to their biology. As much as they may have suffered and as dysfunctional as they may have been with their old ways of thinking about depression, they may have had some continuing illusion of future control stemming from the belief that if they only understood this or changed that, their depression would resolve forever. Toward this end they have persisted and fought. It is true that a biological perspective on depression does underscore a definite vulnerability that will not disappear. However, this is, to the best of our knowledge, the reality. Although the truth will not "set patients free," it will continue to guide them to the most effective means of controlling the disorder and limiting its negative impact on their lives. Patients should *not* infer from it that their best efforts will not matter, or that these efforts will not contribute greatly to their personal well-being.

Psychodynamics of Psychopharmacological Treatment

Involvement in psychopharmacological treatment may have many meanings to those with depression. Therapists employing BIPD must have a thorough comprehension of the psychodynamic forces that are likely to affect patients' willingness to accept and comply with psychopharmacological treatment when it is necessary or desirable. The numerous common obstacles to such treatment must be understood, anticipated, and overcome.

Possibly the most powerful dynamic operating in favor of psychopharmacological treatment is the dynamic of suffering. The inherent anguish of depression and its demoralizing and dysfunctional manifestations drive people to seek help in many different ways: religious and spiritual paths, physical and nutritional regimens, changes in jobs and relationships, sessions with psychics and other parapsychologists, and consultations with mental health professionals of all disciplines. In acute states of depression, people are exceptionally vulnerable; they are often desperate because of multiple failed efforts, and are willing to seek support and hope by any means that seems available to them. All of the approaches mentioned above have advocates offering both hope and support, and undoubtedly some individuals have found benefit from elements of each. With regard to psychopharmacological treatment of depression, both rational and irrational forces may operate to facilitate the treatment: The psychopharmacological approach is supported both by scientific data and by the extensive publicity it has received in the mass media.

Opposing these forces are numerous other psychodynamic forces (Gutheil, 1982), which include resistances based on such personality characteristics as obsessionality, narcissism, passive–aggressive traits, and avoidance. Issues of acceptance and compliance versus resistance and rejection of such treatment are played out around themes of dependency, autonomy, conflicts with authority, and self-esteem. Specific therapeutic approaches utilizing a dynamic understanding of such forces are discussed later in this chapter (see "Psychotherapy in Connection with Psychopharmacological Treatment," below).

Psychodynamics of the Patient–Therapist Relationship

Every treatment relationship within the context of health care contains elements of dependency, authority, mutuality, intimacy, exploration, control, submission, altruism, and numerous other dynamic elements. Clearly, an understanding of these forces by the therapist confers a distinct advantage on the treatment, compared to ignorance of these. These are discussed further in Chapter 6, in the section on "Conduct of the Psychotherapist."

COPING SKILLS EXPLORATION, TRAINING, AND SUPPORT

The concept of "coping" used here incorporates both those psychological homeostatic mechanisms that create the most comfortable internal state for the individual suffering from depression, and those cognitive and behavioral measures that counter the dysfunctional elements of depression. The former occur quite normally and naturally on the basis of trial and error, and depend upon the inclinations of the individual. People who experience emotional pain and turmoil will go to great lengths to discover what makes them feel better, or at least what makes them feel not as bad. They will come to the treatment situation with a broad repertoire of maneuvers both inside their heads and in the world that will limit their pain. Unfortunately, at times these solutions to their pain may result in worsening dysfunction. For instance, individuals may learn that not interacting with others makes them feel less stressed, less irritable, and less self-critical; however, in some situations this primarily adaptive behavior results in poor job performance or absenteeism, which may threaten their livelihood. Strategies for successful coping must therefore take into account both the requirements of the depressed person's emotional suffering and the demands of the world, and must balance these needs.

Coping skills exploration initially involves a systematic inquiry into all of the possible means of coping that patients have utilized in the past or are using currently, as well as an examination of the relative adaptiveness of these methods in balancing the two sets of demands noted above. This search focuses not only on methods of coping that have been employed successfully prior to depression or other crises, but also those that serve the individual on a day-to-day basis in dealing with normal stressors and conflicts. Methods of coping that are beyond the patient's own experiences can be presented by the therapist, who may draw these from his or her own personal and professional experiences, common sense, and the professional literature. The therapist encourages the patient's experimentation with these and supports those reproducible and effective methods that serve to reduce pain, to counter dysfunction, and at times to create positive affect and increase productivity. What are these coping skills? Table 5.2 lists forms of coping that can be explored.

Education

We have already discussed at some length the extraordinarily important elements of coping that are the intellectual and rational processes in-

TABLE 5.2. Forms of Coping to Be Explored with Patients

Education

- Creating rational and intellectual distance from pain
- Understanding depression as an illness
- Limiting dysfunction

Modifying pain

- Suppressing emotions
- Relaxing (through progressive muscle relaxation, autogenic imagery, meditation, or prayer)
- Drawing on spiritual and religious beliefs
- Distracting oneself by active means (cleaning, chores, errands)
- Distracting oneself by passive means (sleeping, TV, music)

Overriding mood

- Exercising strenuously
- Cultivating special relationships
- Enjoying small pleasures
- Relying on the structure of work, home, or school

Transcending cognitive distortions/counteracting moral imperatives

- Identifying distortions and their sources
- Establishing depression's role in distortions
- Reconstructing a "healthier" view
- Recognizing elements of depression that press for harmful action
- Tolerating these elements and persisting in the struggle

Enhancing healthy behavior

- Limiting use of alcohol, caffeine, cigarettes; avoiding substance abuse
- Reducing stressful events

volved with patient education. Such education takes place both in a straightforward scientific manner and through the exploration of the phenomenological and dynamic features that constitute the language of depression. This educational process can diminish pain by creating some emotional distance from it; can afford the depressed patient some mastery of the uncontrolled through understanding; and can limit dysfunction by undermining the moral imperatives of depression's regressive demands. The centrality and importance of education about depression warrant its being dealt with separately, but at its core, such education is a form of coping.

Modifying Pain

Coping mechanisms that modulate the degree of pain include the ability to shut down or constrict affective experience on a conscious level; the capacity through relaxation, guided imagery, or similar techniques to direct one's attention away from the immediate unpleasant experience to another more neutral or even pleasant experience; the ability to achieve comfort or a sense of safety through one's religious and spiritual beliefs and feelings; and the ability to distract oneself from one's immediate state through active efforts to engage in a task or interact with others, or through passive receptivity to the radio, television, or the like.

Overriding Mood

People who have mild to moderate levels of depression may retain the capacity for some pleasures (reactivity). In these circumstances, overcoming depression's barriers to activity—anergy, apathy, fatigue—may actually help such persons to *override* degrees of depressed mood and anhedonia. Behavioral therapies for depression rely on this mechanism to reverse some of the effects and affects of depression. For some patients, running or other strenuous physical activity may improve mood and enhance energy levels, usually on a short-term basis. Special relationships may retain their capacity to provide interest, pleasure, comfort and support. Small pleasures may be obtained from reading, needlepoint, or crossword puzzles.

Employment or school provides structured time, interaction with colleagues, intellectual demands, and a sense of purpose for many who may resist it or wish to withdraw from it. Despite all of the depression-driven problems that can arise in a work or school setting, work or education may also be the most multilevel form of healthy coping available. Even when cognitive functioning is somewhat compromised by the depression, persistence in the workplace or in school is often preferable to the potentially more regressive alternatives.

Transcending Cognitive Distortions/ Counteracting Moral Imperatives

Cognitive skills are employed in formal and specific ways in cognitive therapy for depression as developed by Beck (1976; Beck et al., 1979). Our use of cognitive coping techniques overlaps to some extent with this approach, even though our assumptions about the psychopathology of depression are different. According to Beck's cognitive theory of depression, the basis of psychopathology is distorted thinking, the acquisition of which occurs through development. These distorted and negative views about the self, the world, and the future are seen as causing depression. The treatment of depression consists of a systematic and repetitive challenge to the assumptions behind these negative views, and an active replacement and repetition of positive views that contradict the negative ones. There is a view that people can't "feel bad" if they are "thinking good."

Beck's view of psychopathology is different from the perspective presented here. Although we. agree that many people have acquired elements of negative thinking from many sources (ranging from critical parents to the developmental effects of chronic depression), this negative thinking leads to feelings of unhappiness, self-deprecation, inadequacy, or other forms of transient "upset." As we have said repeatedly, "upset" is not depression, and the bad feelings that people often experience in such circumstances are usually countered quickly by balancing views. This is a coping mechanism that occurs naturally and normally with the development of cognitive abilities. Most nondepressed people are exposed to transient narcissistic injuries every day of their lives, and rather quickly dispose of their potential upset through numerous face-saving and esteem-building mechanisms, including rationalization ("I only got a B because I didn't try hard enough"), identification ("So I didn't get promoted—my Bears are still the champs"), devaluation ("Who cares if she didn't say 'Hello'—she's a Methodist"), and idealization ("No matter what happens, my mother [or God] loves me"). In nondepressed people, these mechanisms work even when there are deep-seated problems with self-esteem, and even in cases where disapproving others think that the people *should* suffer more!

The failure of these mechanisms in depression is a product of the depression. Depressed mood and impairment in the functioning of the pleasure center are what primarily drive the distorted thinking. Once the thinking is negative, it only serves to aggravate and deepen the depression; this vicious cycle is what creates the moral imperative to move toward regressive, maladaptive, and potentially destructive consequences. For these reasons, the employment of cognitive techniques becomes an important part of coping with depression. In conjunction with other elements of treatment, cognitive methods have clearly demonstrated their efficacy in mild to moderate depression.

BIPD generally assumes that regressive cognitive distortions arise from four sources: universal developmental dynamics (with their idiosyncratic corollaries); the vicissitudes of life; amplification of depression-driven functional impairments; and depression's power to tip the scales of perception in the most negative direction. Therapeutic strategies for dealing with cognitive distortions in depression should include the following:

1. Identifying each distortion and its source.
2. Establishing the role of depression in precipitating or emphasizing the negative perception.
3. Reconstructing a "balanced" view that reflects the truer self.

An example demonstrates the use of these strategies.

> Following a minor setback at work, a depressed business executive became preoccupied with his personal failings, his inability to succeed, and the hopelessness of even making a sustained effort. In exploring the sources of such feelings, he described the many circumstances in which he was unable to compete successfully with his older brothers, leaving him feeling ashamed and inadequate. As a means of compensation, he became a tenacious competitor—an overachiever who accomplished a great deal more than he expected. When he was not depressed, he took on any setback as a further challenge and dug in harder. When he was depressed, these developmental themes joined forces with his immediate disappointments to create a powerful regressive state. When it was pointed out how his depression was driving the regression, he could see it intellectually, but persisted in feeling defeated. However, with repeated similar experiences, he was able to transcend the way he felt and to act not upon his perceived failure, but upon his knowledge that this state was temporary and would change as his depression lifted. He could therefore act "as if" he were his usual self. Such a response might or might not have an effect on his mood, but it at least alleviated some of his sense of helplessness, as well as whatever pressure he felt about quitting his job.

It is important to appreciate that although the application of all of these cognitive coping skills remains wise in more severe depressions (and even some less severe depressions), the power of such depressions may be sufficient to prevent patients from using these skills or to minimize their impact. At such times, only treatment with antidepressant medication may alleviate the depression sufficiently for patients to be able to take advantage of these other measures.

As a product of the cognitive distortions of depression, the "moral imperatives" of depression become special targets of coping skills training and therapeutic intervention. The three moral imperatives that are most seductive, and at the same time destructive, to depressed patients are those to end relationships, to quit work, or to kill themselves. (Suicide, the third element of this triad, is addressed separately later in this chapter.) Each of these may seem like the only way out of pain at the time, but each ultimately undermines patients' future functioning or lives. Being able to recognize when the "depression is talking" can be a critical skill that helps the individuals prevent the subverting effects of their depression.

Although some marriages, friendships, and other relationships may be able to tolerate depressed persons' acting upon their internal experiences and distortions, over time such actions will erode the quality of these relationships. The decision to end a relationship on the basis of imbalanced depressive perceptions may be "reversible" in some instances, but such decisions are likely to lead over time to increasing isolation and lack of support. Similarly, careers and jobs are not easily established or maintained under the best of circumstances. People whose depressive experiences lead them to withdraw from or reject their work not only risk the immediate consequences, but, more importantly, may develop a trend (albeit a well-rationalized one) of downward mobility. Given the centrality of relationships and work within all of our lives, and perhaps the even greater importance of these for those who are depressed, there are few more crucial elements of psychotherapy on the part of either patients or therapists than the fight against the moral imperatives that undermine these areas of life.

The coping skills that are essential for patients to learn are the abilities to recognize and to tolerate those elements of depression pressing for action that may be harmful to their relationships or work. Recognition, in particular, involves the heightening of patients' self-consciousness and skepticism about the validity of their perceptions. A parallel process should be occurring in therapists as well; in fact, a therapist may need to develop this skepticism first and teach it to a patient. This is a difficult task for both therapist and patient. For the therapist, it will involve modification of a basically empathic and accepting stance. For both therapist and patient, it will require the adoption of doubt and skepticism in dealing with a person who is already self-deprecating and often doubting of his or her most fundamental personal beliefs. On the surface of things, such an approach would seem to make matters worse for the patient: "I'm already suffering. Why can't I at least act upon the feelings I have? Why should I be made to feel more incompetent?" On the other hand, an understanding of depression makes it clear that depression-driven actions will lead to further loss and deterioration. The therapist who remains unequivocally empathic only reinforces the depressed patient's maladaptive distortions and rationalizations.

A therapist's activity is often necessary for a patient to counteract the moral imperatives of depression. Even experienced and skilled psychotherapists may have difficulty convincing given depressed patients that they are acting under the influence of depression. However, if therapists do not attempt to convince patients of this—even to the extent of "fighting" with patients if necessary—the patients are much more likely to succumb and further complicate their lives. Over time, most such patients will come to incorporate the therapists' perspective: to recognize the language of their depression; to tolerate the pressure to act upon these distortions; and to persist in their struggles to maintain their relationships and/or work.

These considerations do not preclude the possibility that a depressed individual may be in a "bad" relationship or the "wrong" job. The exploration of such possibilities ought to occur, however, at a time when the individual's mood is sufficiently stable that depression is not "running the show."

Enhancing Healthy Behavior

Although many coping skills are effective in both raising the threshold of pain and not interfering with adaptive functioning or even facilitating such functioning, many others help people feel better but are otherwise maladaptive. Alcohol and other central nervous system depressants, though at times effective for short-term mood elevation or "numbing" of emotional pain, can worsen depression, compromise health, and impair judgment over time. Stimulants (amphetamines, cocaine), marijuana, and hallucinogens are "beneficial" as short-term mood elevators, and marijuana can also settle the irritability of depression, but all can create other psychiatric and legal complications with prolonged use. Similarly, some depressed patients will discover that food, sex, cigarettes, and spending money provide short-term relief and long-term maladaptive consequences. The therapeutic tasks in such situations include empathic exploration and appreciation of the important roles that such behaviors have provided in helping the depressed patients to manage painful or unbearable affects, as well as helping the patients to understand the potential destructiveness of each of these behaviors. Whenever other, healthier coping skills (e.g., avoidance or reduction of stressful events) can be employed, they should be encouraged and supported. When affects remain unbearable, more aggressive psychopharmacological management should be employed.

General Comments

In traditional insight-oriented therapies, the therapist's involvement with coping skills exploration, training, or support has been demeaned because such activity does not lead to "cure" (as it has been assumed that only uncovering and understanding do). Such approaches have also been thought to interfere with the development of the transference neurosis by "distorting" the role of the therapist and by satisfying rather than frustrating patients' needs, further blocking the ultimate goal of knowledge.

Employment of coping techniques involves the recognition that depression has no cure. At best, depression can be controlled and its impact minimized. Coping should be seen not only as honorable and legitimate, but as *optimal* in terms of our current understanding of depressive disorders and the psychotherapeutic approaches to them.

WORK WITH SIGNIFICANT OTHERS

The impact of a person's depression seldom escapes those around him or her. Family and friends often see the person's suffering and may bear the brunt of some of it. Engaging important family members (especially a spouse, parents, or children living in the same home as the depressed person) in the therapeutic work can be quite helpful to both the patient and the family members in a number of ways. Work with significant others may include some or all of the following:

1. Assessment
2. Education
3. Support
4. Treatment of relationship problems
5. Monitoring

Assessment

Although nearly all depressed people can identify that they are suffering in a variety of ways (i.e., they can subjectively describe their symptoms), they may not recognize the effects they may be having on their families. It's easy for people to realize that they are not sleeping well, or feeling tired, slowed down, unhappy, angry, or painfully sad. However, those who are depressed are often preoccupied, overly self-absorbed, or so "captured" by the depression that they have lost the capacity to see how they are affecting those around them. When a patient is married or involved in a long-term relationship, input from the spouse or partner may deepen both the therapist's and the patient's understanding of the depression and its impact. Parents can provide developmental data that may be inaccessible to the patient; information about genetic contributions to a depressive diathesis is thus more likely to be complete, and parental observations about early-life manifestations of depression can help to clarify its course. Lingering notions from traditional treatments of depression that the patient's recollections and impressions are of paramount importance must sometimes give way to the need for firmer data, which at times only others can provide.

Education

The family members' needs to understand the nature, impact, and language of depression are often as great as the patient's. Involving significant others, especially a spouse or partner, in this process should occur early in the treatment. Like the patient, family members should be given a "spiel" explaining what is known about depression, and should be encouraged to do independent reading; the same bibliography can be used.

Exploration of the language of depression, especially as it pertains to a marriage or a similar relationship, ought to occur in the presence of both the patient and the spouse or partner for several reasons. The effects of depression on the relationship may be subtle or blatant: reflections of the patient's heightened sensitivity and vulnerability, greater irritability, a tendency to withdraw, a lack of interest in sex or perhaps anything, criticisms about "old issues" that had been dormant, an intense neediness that elicits rejection, or many other problems. Effective exploration requires identification of the issues, direct feedback about the ways they are manifested, descriptions of their impact and the interactions they stimulate, and each partner's interpretations of them. The therapist can help both partners by providing a model for how to proceed—having sufficient objectivity to demonstrate respect for each person's perspective, while helping both to understand that substantial elements of such problematic interactions are direct products of depression. The therapist's stance of interpreting these potentially volatile experiences as "artifacts" teaches the couple this perspective. With both partners present and actively responding, the education comes alive. Any criticisms, distortions and misattributions that arise can be dealt with immediately.

Support

As the depressed person and the spouse or partner, for example, learn the language of depression as it appears in their relationship, there is often a shift in both of their perspectives, especially in regard to their attributions of the meanings of difficult interactions. A wife who has interpreted her husband's sullen withdrawal as a primary comment on their relationship or a criticism of her can come to appreciate that this is "the depression talking." She can transcend her automatic responses of hurt and anger (which, with repeated reattribution, may recede), and can approach him in an empathic or sympathetic and supportive way. This is the same principle that we have described repeatedly: Once a phenomenon has been reinterpreted as an artifact of depression, its legitimacy is undermined, and the moral imperative to respond to it as legitimate is also undermined. Instead of seeing such interactions as inflammatory, both the patient and the spouse or partner come to see these as depression-driven and state-dependent behaviors and issues. This approach thus enables the nondepressed partner to recognize manifestations of depression, sidestep conflict, and offer support.

> When Phyllis became depressed, her withdrawal and lack of sexual interest left Roger feeling rejected, annoyed, and helpless. His efforts to soothe her were met with unresponsiveness from Phyllis. His subsequent annoyance and suggestions that she "snap out of it" left Phyllis feeling even worse. When Phyllis's depression was identified as something that victimized her as well as Roger, he was able to disengage from his perception of an interpersonal struggle between them. Phyllis still suffered, as did Roger, but Roger was able to ally himself with her against a common enemy until her depression lifted. He was able to see that he neither caused the problem nor had the power to fix it, but could only understand it and empathize with Phyllis's plight. Her behavior, though superficially appearing to be a rejection of him, was primarily a product of her depression; it thus became more tolerable to him.

Once a particular depression-related interpersonal problem has been identified as such, a couple or family may discuss how to anticipate future recurrences. What response will be most appreciated by, or simply acceptable to, the depressed person in the throes of a negative mood? An empathic comment? A hug without words? Avoidance? At the very least, there is likely to be a recognition that processing the conflict may be impossible or undesirable while the depressed person is experiencing a distortion, exaggeration of affect, or general regression. An agreement about how the couple or family should proceed may not solve the "crisis," but it may limit the relationship deterioration that may have been a consequence in the past.

Treatment of Relationship Problems

Although work with couples (and families) in which one member is depressed tends to focus on the impact of the depression on their lives, there is a risk of their developing an inclination to see *all* difficult behavior or interaction as being simply depression-driven. A lack of balance and appreciation for the complexity of such phenomena can lead to the depressed person's being seen as someone without any legitimate complaints or feelings, but as someone who is defined by the depression. This can be demeaning and demoralizing, especially for someone who may already feel inadequate for being depressed and impaired. A given complaint or criticism may be driven by depression and magnified by this state, but it will often have roots in the ambivalence and conflict that exist in normal living.

All relationships contain degrees of ambivalence and personal differences in communications, style, aesthetics, beliefs, and goals. Effective relationships can be achieved on the one hand through open expressions of these, with negotiation and compromise toward a mutually "fair" settlement; or, on the other hand, through the use of varying degrees of denial, acceptance, patience, and forgiveness for areas of persistent disagreement. These accommodations may lead to a general state of satisfaction and a "good enough" personality in an individual. When depression occurs, there will be state-dependent regressions that will aggravate and intensify such ambivalence and differences, making them appear pathological and unworkable. At times, this process may lead to an apparent "existential crisis" in a relationship, threatening its existence.

As in work with a depressed individual, the therapist working with such a couple when such state-dependent regression is occurring should not overstate pathology within the relationship. Efforts to determine the stable configuration of conflicts and problems may be possible through retrospective assessment of the relationship. More often, though, this process is colored by the impact of depression on both people. Much as in individual work, the therapist's task is to help the couple identify elements of depression, cope with and limit the damage, and reassess the relationship for ongoing problems once the affective episode has stabilized. If there are important long-standing conflicts to be dealt with and both partners have an interest in proceeding with these, couple therapy may be optional. If it becomes clear that primary relationship issues are contributing as stressors to the precipitation or aggravation of depressive episodes, such treatment will be desirable. However, there should be no *a priori* assumptions that relationship problems are contributory simply because they are expressed as depressive phenomena.

> When Dave's mood was stable, he and Sandy were at peaceful odds about differences in their personal styles. Dave was quite fastidious, but had become tolerant of Sandy's "relaxed" ways about their home. Although he did not quite find these endearing, he saw with amusement their idiosyncrasies as human foibles. When depressive periods emerged, however, Dave found himself increasingly intolerant of the "mess" he had to endure, eventually engaging in a merciless diatribe against Sandy, "the spoiled bitch" who was deliberately upsetting him with her filth.

The effects of the depression seemed to intensify Dave's compulsivity while simultaneously diminishing his tolerance for Sandy's stance. His hostility and sense of entitlement to express it resulted in devastating attacks upon his wife. Sandy developed an appreciation for the language of Dave's depression that helped her detach somewhat from such attacks. During Dave's periods of remission, they were able to return to their struggle as a couple to reconcile this disparity. Each could see the legitimacy of the other's perspective, and Dave could acknowledge that he "got crazy" about this during his depression. Repeated experiences with this issue eventually enabled Dave to contain his intensifying feelings even when he was depressed.

Regardless of the presence or absence of "baseline" pathology in the relationship, there is usually some "cleanup" work to be done by the couple (in or out of formal therapy) following a depressive episode. It is usually helpful for the couple to look back at such an episode with the therapist, to develop a method of reviewing how each party handled the experience, and to explore residual damage (anger, demoralization, embarrassment).

With each depressive episode, Ted focused his anger upon Kim. Prior to treatment, these bursts of anger escalated quickly to name calling and the physical destruction of property, with threats of personal violence. Kim's efforts to calm Ted were met with escalation of his rage, and Kim learned over time to stay away. When the depression and rage subsided, Ted was too embarrassed to acknowledge his behavior or apologize; his embarrassment only contributed further to a residue of resentment at Kim for being a witness to his disgrace. Kim, thankful only that the rage had passed, was too frightened to address these issues, so that a history of unresolved experiences built up. Once Ted entered treatment, antidepressants helped to diminish the frequency and intensity of his angry episodes. As Ted identified his rage toward Kim as an artifact of his depression, it undermined the legitimacy and frequency of his acting out.

In couple therapy, Kim was able to talk about her fears of Ted's rage and the paralysis it created in her. Ted experienced great remorse and was able to apologize to Kim both in sessions and whenever he was caught up in what were their less intense episodes. At such times, he was increasingly able to contain his feelings. He came to understand that his view of a woman's role was to protect him from harm and soothe away pain, and that, unrealistic as this expectation may have been, his resentment was based on depressive pain from which Kim could not save him. When Ted was in remission, he and Kim agreed that the fundamental structure of their relationship was a good one and that their primary need as a couple was for mutual protection from Ted's depression.

Monitoring

Work with significant others can at times incorporate family members as part of a treatment "team" in the sense that they may take on the role of monitors. In most relationships, this monitoring function takes the form of regular feedback—for example, feedback from a nondepressed spouse or partner to a depressed one about what he or she has observed and how the depression seems to manifest itself. Further feedback from the depressed person is then invited. In this form, monitoring helps both parties watch more carefully for depressive manifestations.

However, monitoring may become part of a safety net for a patient whose depressive episodes are sufficiently severe to warrant identifying others besides the patient and therapist as agents of communication to the therapist. This may occur under circumstances when a patient is sufficiently consumed by the disorder to be unable to judge accurately what is happening to him or her, and/or under circumstances of great risk.

It has become common practice to establish a network of supportive family members, friends, employers, caseworkers, and even conservators to operate as monitors for many patients with potential psychotic disorders such as schizophrenia or for patients with recurrent mania. This becomes more complicated with depressed patients, because of the great degree of variability of risk and the inherently patronizing aspects of being someone's monitor. Monitoring assumes issues of authority and control that would normally not be granted to another adult. At times, this situation feels like a further assault on a patient's sense of autonomy, which has already been undermined by this illness. On the other hand, it is a reality that depression does have the capacity to strip the healthiest of people of their critical judgment and perspective, putting them at great risk.

Patients and their families are often torn by their ambivalence about having others (including a therapist) enter into a monitoring role. No one wants to infantilize patients unnecessarily, but everyone wants them to be safe. Overprotective loved ones may move too quickly, civil libertarians too late. This problem needs to be discussed extensively with every patient and family, and all parties need to reach an understanding of how communications between family and therapist will be handled. The issues include not only confidentiality (which must be defined), but also the question of when to act. Certainly therapists must be able to receive and act upon all information pertinent to suicide (see the discussion of this topic later in this chapter). Most families who become worried about their loved ones' deterioration will communicate apparent suicidal intent to the therapist, regardless of what has previously been decided. As a result, therapists and patients with the best of plans may find themselves doing "cleanup" work—that is, having to process what seem like violations of patients' confidentiality.

> Rebecca's relationship with her mother was almost always predictably state-dependent. When she was stable, she felt quite autonomous and could interact with her mother with amicable distance. When she was depressed, Rebecca became intensely dependent and rejection-sensitive, desperate for her mother's support, and easily deflated by any hesitancy on the part of this naturally reserved woman. When she was euthymic, Rebecca refused to have her therapist talk with her mother; when she was depressed, she frightened her mother sufficiently to precipitate a call to the therapist pleading for help for both of them. Each time this occurred, Rebecca and the therapist struggled with the reality that she was different people at different times with different needs. She would be angry that her autonomy had been breached by these communications between her mother and therapist, but she ultimately recognized (once she was euthymic) that the regression of her illness forced such contact, and that neither her mother nor her therapist could ignore her "cry for help."

This example also highlights an apparent paradox of treatment planning: It too is state-dependent, and flexible guidelines are necessary. With regard to the use of significant others for reporting to either patient or therapist, the overriding principle is to preserve the patient's safety whenever necessary and to preserve his or her autonomy whenever possible.

PSYCHOTHERAPY IN CONNECTION WITH PSYCHOPHARMACOLOGICAL TREATMENT

Psychopharmacological treatment of depression, especially moderate and severe depression, has become standard in the United States over the past decade. In many centers, including our own, even mild depressions that exhibit automony and persistence over time are treated aggressively with antidepressant medication. The use of medication in conjunction with psychotherapy has been shown to be a highly effective approach to treating the depressive disorders (Elkin et al., 1989; Kupfer et al., 1992; Rush et al., 1977). Yet depression continues to be underdiagnosed, and even when diagnosed to be untreated or undertreated (Roberts & Vernon, 1982).

In 1990, the NIMH developed the Depression Awareness, Recognition and Treatment (DART) Program. This is a nationwide program aimed at greater public and professional education about the depressive disorders and their treatment. We are beginning to see the effects of such efforts at public education and of mass media exposure, as more and more patients present themselves after reading about depression in the newspaper or watching a television show about it. However, many patients and clinical practitioners continue to be reluctant to utilize psychopharmacological agents, either alone or in conjunction with psychotherapy. Let us consider this resistance, first as it occurs in professionals and then in patients.

Psychotherapists' Resistance to Psychopharmacology

Psychotherapists' reluctance to employ medication in the treatment of depression has its roots in traditional beliefs about the nature of psychopathology and the central role of psychotherapy as the ultimate curative agent. Even when there was empirical evidence of the effectiveness of antidepressant medications, there was a view that "resorting" to pharmacology was evidence of failure in the psychotherapy or a manifestation of therapist frustration or other countertransference problems. This view was fairly standard in the 1950s and 1960s, when psychoanalytic philosophy and training dominated U.S. psychiatry. Klerman (1984), in discussing the pros and cons of the combined use of psychotherapy and psychopharmacology, has described this historical perspective. Traditionalists cited, and in some cases continue to cite, a number of arguments supporting the belief that drugs interfere with the treatment of depression (Rounsaville et al., 1981).

The following points draw upon Klerman's (1984) observations and address them from our perspective.

1. *Drug treatment introduces a placebo effect. The symbolic meaning of being given a pill promotes the authoritarian elements of treatment and heightens a patient's dependency and magical expectations.* In fact, these concerns are legitimate. To the extent that pharmacological treatment often has a dramatic and "magical" quality in resolving depression and relieving suffering, this quality may become the rationale for its use. The efficacy of antidepressant treatment and the expertise of the treater do undermine the egalitarianism to which traditional therapy aspires. On the other hand, all of our knowledge of transference leads us to the conclusion that such aspirations have always been illusory; concerns about the inherent dependency fostered by effective treatment are applicable to many other aspects of the therapist–patient relationship. These concerns should be translated into efforts to limit dependency and to promote patient autonomy through other means (to be described below).

2. *Drug therapy reduces patients' anxiety, depression, and other symptoms, and thereby diminishes their motivation for psychotherapy.* The traditioinal view is that most people suffer from "neuroses" in a fundamental way, and that psychotherapy is necessary or at least desirable for everyone. The "ticket of admission" to treatment is often a crisis or a particular set of symptoms; however, it is understood that the crisis or symptoms are only surface manifestations of deeper levels of pathology, which require analytic psychotherapy. Because distress and symptoms may be transient and tend to resolve spontaneously, leading to a "flight into health" (i.e., patients feel better and do not think they need further treatment), traditional therapists' efforts to overcome patients' resistance and intensify their motivation for treatment consist of making ego-dystonic what is ego-syntonic. That is, "striking while the iron is hot," or when patients are still in distress, involves uncovering old wounds, eliciting the universally unresolved conflicts of childhood and latent impediments to self-esteem, and creating an understanding of still-extant psychopathology that needs work. Suffering provides the early motivation for such treatment, and removing the suffering with medication does undermine the process. This would indeed be detrimental if there were any substantial evidence that the underlying pathology is known or that the traditional form of treatment is curative, protective, or even related to the actual caues of depression.

On the contrary, we believe that psychotherapeutic techniques for the treatment of symptomatic disorders in general, and certainly for the treatment of depression, should be anxiety-reducing. There are already significant elements of anxiety introduced by the depression itself, as well as by the problems that the depression creates. Furthermore, elevating anxiety is likely to exacerbate or exaggerate depressive symptoms.

3. *Psychopharmacology may have a negative effect by undercutting the patient's defenses and causing symptom substitution.* This objection is based on the view that there is a dynamic balance of ego-defensive operations, a kind of "hydraulic model" of psychopathology: If pressure is removed from one place, it will show up elsewhere. This argument has been used against behavioral therapies and has shown no validity in that context. Studies of psychopharmacological treatment have also failed to demonstrate this; in other words, successful treatment has been successful.

4. *Psychopharmacological treatment may have a deleterious effect because some patients will see their treatment with medicine as evidence that they are "sicker" than patients who only need psychotherapy.* This argument may seem particularly valid if one believes in the value of insight as curative. From this perspective, patients receiving medication may see themselves as less "worthy" and less interesting to the therapist. Of course,

this view should be modified by a change in patients' and therapists' understanding of psychopathology.

All of these concerns have influenced, and to a certain extent continue to influence, the attitudes and beliefs of psychotherapists in regard to the use of antidepressants. Other issues may also contribute to therapists' resistance to incorporating psychopharmacological treatment. Many clinicians have difficulty in accepting a biological framework that challenges the traditional view of pathology. Not only may they find these concepts less intellectually stimulating, but they may be reluctant to abandon long-standing and hard-won beliefs. Moreover, if therapists are not physicians, they may see their own efforts as devalued in comparison to pharmacological treatment. A psychotherapy focused more on coping than on cure may also be inherently less appealing. Finally, some therapists may have struggled through their own depressions without pharmacological intervention, and may thus be convinced that whatever treatment they had was correct; other therapists may have been treated with antidepressant medication, but ineffectively, insufficiently, or with complications. All of these factors may contribute to a bias against psychopharmacology.

The effectiveness of integrated treatment depends upon the consistency and agreement of the members of the treatment team in cases where the roles of psychotherapist and psychopharmacologist are split, or upon the internal consistency of the psychiatrist/psychotherapist who is playing both roles. Although the efficacy of psychopharmacological treatment does not rely on the convictions of either patient or therapist, it does depend upon patients' availability for continuous or intermittent pharmacotherapy, and certainly patients are less likely to make themselves available for such treatment if their therapists are not convinced of its importance (although there are many patients who recognize antidepressants as essential to their well-being, in the face of indifference or opposition from their psychotherapists).

Over time, there has been a gradual erosion of therapists' strict adherence to psychoanalytically oriented views. Several forces have contributed to this change:

1. *Practical considerations.* Few people can afford, and few insurance policies pay for, intensive long-term treatment. This has forced therapists to abbreviate and modify their treatment approaches.

2. *Research and training in new psychotherapeutic approaches* (specifically CBT and IPT). The proven efficacy of such treatments, particularly in the short-term treatment of depression, has resulted in the incorporation of many of their elements into this work.

3. *The efficacy of psychopharmacology.* Aside from the research data, clinicians are usually only convinced of the power of antidepressants after they have seen them work.

4. *Increasing understanding of the biology of depression.* This provides a strong rationale to support biological treatments and at times to de-emphasize psychological approaches, particularly in those patients with extensive family histories of depression and minimal previous responses to psychotherapeutic interventions.

5. *Changes within the field of psychoanalysis.* The "movement" has lost many of its most conservative adherents, and members of the newer breed of clinicians gravitating toward psychoanalytic work are often grounded in current biological theories; the field is thus becoming more flexible.

Despite these trends, a strong residue of traditional thinking about symptomatic psychopathology exists among clinicians and the culture as a whole, and this view tends to create resistance to pharmacological treatment. In clinicians, this may take the form of reluctant permission for their patients to try antidepressants, rather than wholehearted endorsement of and commitment to such treatment. When patients express resistance, do not respond to the first intervention, or have some problems with side effects, such therapists will be too ready to "pull the plug" on such treatment, reinforce the patients' resistance, and resume a psychotherapy-only approach. Overcoming this resistance requires a continuing systematic identification and challenge of such clinicians' underlying attitudes and beliefs about psychopathology and psychopharmacology. These same principles also apply to patients' resistance.

Patients' Resistance to Psychopharmacology

The reluctance of patients to utilize psychopharmacological treatment for depression often parallels that of therapists. We all live in the same culture, which idealizes, promotes, and rewards self-sufficiency. We all recognize as healthy the inclination to seek mastery and achieve control within our personal lives. Such personal philosophies guide the lives of our most successful people, and most of us are generally unwilling to compromise our sense of autonomy and personal control, except under extraordinary circumstances. As powerful as such forces are in a general sense, they are much more so when we are dealing with the possibility of giving someone else the control of our brain functions.

People are quite willing to use nicotine, alcohol, and many other mind-altering drugs when they have control—or at least the illusion of control—over how they utilize them. Inviting others, even generally trusted professionals (which psychiatrists and other physicians may not always be), to give them pills that will alter the chemical composition of their brains is not a concept individuals readily embrace. It takes considerable suffering to overcome this resistance. In addition, it takes education to appreciate the full implications of the disorder for which a drug is being used, the properties of the drug, and the kinds of problems and responses that can be expected. As is often the case with therapists, patients who are depressed tend to see their depressions in existential terms, often subscribe to traditional views of underlying causes, and wish to "talk their way" or "love their way" out of their depressions.

Helping Patients to Accept and Continue Psychopharmacological Treatment

Central to pharmacological treatment is educating patients about what we know of this disorder: its description, various manifestations, and language; its prevalence; its biological elements, including genetics; and psychological factors that may contribute to its expression and that are likely to be affected by it. This information should be presented authoritatively, and as much of the patients' own experience as possible should be incorporated into the presentation. Patients and their significant others should be encouraged to read in as much detail as possible, with as scientific an orientation as they may be capable of, and to whatever extent is necessary to inform them fully about what is wrong, what treatments are available, and what the range of outcomes may be. In addition, when pharmacological treatment of the depression is indicated, therapists should anticipate the common kinds of resistance to pharmacological treatment and make specific inquiries about the patients' possible hesitancy and concerns, addressing whatever issues may arise in the fashion described in this book.

This is a very active process of inquiry and reeducation; the persistence and perseverance with which a therapist pursues it depend upon and are in proportion to the severity of a patient's depression. The therapist needs to be unrelenting and yet quite empathic in the face of the patient's possible ignorance, fears, and refusal to relinquish control. The driving forces behind these efforts to "sell" pharmacological treatment are the therapist's recognition of the patient's suffering and his or her knowledge of and conviction about the therapeutic efficacy of antidepressants. Such a stance is necessary for both the physician prescribing antidepressants and the nonphysician psychotherapist who are working together. The more people who can support a consistent and well-informed view of this treatment, the easier it will be for the patient to maintain.

When patients are suffering, they are often more open to accepting the views, the help, and the medicine of others than when they are "themselves." When depression remits or is controlled and patients regain their premorbid status, most experience a profound sense of relief, as well as a deepened appreciation of their therapists' knowledge and the treatment's effectiveness. Their recovery is the confirmation of the educational process, and will serve as encouragement to follow through with whatever treatment plan has been developed (even though their "single-sample studies" have no scientific validity). Some patients, however, respond to their recovery with denial. Their illness, their regression, and their compromised functioning have seemingly made them so vulnerable that they cannot accept any view of themselves that includes the continuing possibility of recurrence. Such people will ascribe their depression to any circumstances over which they believe they have achieved control. They are likely to discontinue antidepressants, insisting that their recovery is something they have accomplished on their own (albeit with some temporary support) and that the medications have played no part in it. Occasionally, these individuals will be spared from learning the full truth and will have no recurrence. However, there is a high probability that within days, weeks, or months of discontinuing antidepressants, the depression will become worse or recur. This process may repeat itself until such a patient overcomes the denial (i.e., the patient's "single-sample study with a crossover design" is valid) or the depression remits permanently.

At the start of therapy, patients' compliance with antidepressant treatment is a function of education and trust. Continued compliance, however, depends on tolerance and efficacy. Antidepressant medications, though generally among the safer drugs in the physician's arsenal, do have a host of side effects; these may range from nuisances to factors prohibiting continued treatment. More serious side effects (e.g., altered cardiac conduction and contractility, seizures, blood dyscrasias, etc.) clearly require close monitoring and supervision by internists, cardiologists, and other specialists. However, most of the side effects can be monitored and care supervised by the psychiatrist. Psychiatrists are required to know the wide variety of side effects, including dry mouth, blurred vision, lightheadedness, constipation or diarrhea, irregular heartbeats, urinary retention, agitation or sedation, nervousness or sleeplessness, weight gain, or any of a number of sexual function disturbances (changes in libido, erectile and ejaculatory dysfunctions, and many more). Nonphysician therapists should develop a general familiarity with the profiles of side effects associated with the major classes of drugs used in the treatment of depression: SSRIs and nonselective monoamine uptake inhibitors, MAOIs, atypical agents, mood stabilizers, anxiolytics, psychostimulants, hormones, and so forth (see Chapter 1). Helping patients to separate side effects from symptoms of their depression or possible medical disorders about which they may be concerned is an important ongoing task, for which information from multiple sources may be useful.

Patients will learn about side effects from their therapists and other physicians, from reading, and from their personal experiences. Personal experience is the most powerful teacher but can also be quite disconcerting and frightening, even when patients are well educated about such effects. The ignorance, lack of control, and fear will at times converge; as a result, patients may come to believe that they have serious medical problems, that they are not good candidates for antidepressant treatment, or at the very least that they should stop their treatment temporarily. For these reasons, part of the process of educating patients involves inquiring about new or worrisome side effects. A few minutes of telephone conversation will usually result in rather immediate reassurance or some minor adjustments that will make continued treatment possible. This approach is far preferable to the patient's stoically accepting side effects (which on rare occasions can have serious consequences), stopping the treatment in order to wait for the next appointment safely, or losing the motivation for treatment because of repeated episodes of side effects that are more prolonged than necessary.

Treating Refractory Depression

What happens if antidepressant treatment is unsuccessful? From a psychopharmacological standpoint, there are numerous strategies for treating refractory depressions (Nierenberg & White, 1990). These include changing from one class of drug to another; augmenting primary antidepressants with lithium carbonate, thyroid hormones, or amphetamines; or combining different classes of antidepressant medications. Usually held in reserve is the use of ECT, although this safe, quick, and effective treatment may be used earlier for psychotically depressed patients or for elderly patients with medical contraindications to antidepressants. Other biological alternatives include bright light treatment and sleep deprivation, but their use in clinical practice has not yet become routine. Although our focus is not on specific psychopharmacological interventions, it is important to note that there are a great many options currently available and that still more new drugs are being developed for the future. Furthermore, it is now known that many patients who have not responded to the first 10 approaches have responded to the 11th. Eight out of 10 patients should achieve full or at least partial "recovery" from an acute episode with aggressive treatment.

From a psychotherapeutic standpoint, the tasks of the therapist

working with a refractory patient include (aside from any other therapeutic maneuvers) helping the patient cope with repeated failures, combat demoralization, and maintain sufficient hope and persistence to stay
the course rather than give up on treatment or life. The therapist must
guard against the effects of his or her own disappointment, frustration,
and demoralization—inevitable consequences when one is treating a
refractory depression. An all-too-common, understandable, but unacceptable response of therapists in such situations is to blame the victims:
"She is resistant," "He doesn't really want to get better," "She enjoys
suffering," or our favorite, "Too much secondary gain." These comments
are the psychological and moral equivalents of "We really pander too
much to those people with cerebral palsy," or "He was trying to get cancer." Such views represent both the loss of empathy born of therapists'
frustration and intolerance of their own helplessness, and the most destructive perversion of psychological attribution.

Therapists, patients, and family members alike frequently lose sight
of the persistent reality that *depression is the enemy*. When this occurs,
everyone gets blamed: Therapists aren't smart enough, don't care enough,
or are simply money-grubbers; patients don't try hard enough, choose
illness, or enjoy suffering; and significant others are selfish, unfeeling, or
hostile. In reality, chronic unremitting depression produces inexorable
anguish, robs its victims of their lives, and torments everyone else who
cares about the sufferers. There is no psychological mechanism compat-
ible with human adaptation that would "choose" such suffering; there is
no amount of secondary gain that could approach logarithmically the
profundity of the primary loss. Yet, once again, these perspectives are
central to traditional views of unconscious motivational factors, as well
as their translation into popular views of individuals' ultimate control
over their lives. The continued propagation of such concepts has many
destructive consequences, including the "justifiable" abandonment of
victims by their families, the disruption of the therapeutic alliance, and
the addition of another layer of suffering (self-blame) to those in need
of greater patience and relief.

If patients have been unable to find effective treatment for their
depression, this is simply a tragedy for them and their families, and a
source of distress for those who are treating them. Because therapists
have greater distance from the suffering and should understand the
all-too-human inclinations toward self-protection, they must not only
recognize these phenomena for what they are, but even anticipate their
appearance and prepare patients, families, and themselves for this. A
therapist treating a patient whose depression is refractory will need to
confront these issues repeatedly and consistently, neither blaming or
abandoning the patient. On the contrary, it is critical for the therapist

to acknowledge how difficult it is for the patient to face the consequences of his or her illness every day; how inclined to lose hope the patient may be in such circumstances; how there is an inevitable wish to be saved from this fate by death or suicide; and how the frustration and disappointment may be turned toward those closest to the patient. Having examined these painful realities with the patient, the therapist must still find hope and convey this to the patient—hope that the introduction of a new pharmacotherapeutic regimen will be effective (which it may), and hope that some means of coping that has not yet worked may soon do so, in order to make life more bearable.

For the psychiatrist treating the patient with refractory depression, a number of considerations are worth reviewing. We call these "the six D's."

1. *Diagnosis.* The psychiatrist should review findings and extend the workup to be sure the patient does not have another treatable primary medical disorder, bipolarity, psychosis, or an anxiety disorder. Similarly, the patient may have a particular subtype of depression that requires a specific approach, such as an MAOI for atypical depression or light treatment for a seasonal mood disorder.

2. *Dose.* The psychiatrist should make sure that the amount of an antidepressant is sufficient. Idiosyncratic variations of metabolism can result in up to 40-fold differences in the effective doses for individuals (Preskorn & Fast, 1991; Schatzberg, 1991).

3. *Duration.* Beliefs about the adequacy of time on an effective dose have been evolving toward persisting with a given drug for up to 2–3 months to obtain optimum results (Prien & Kupfer, 1986; Quitkin et al., 1984).

4. *Drug changes.* Often, switching from one class to another is more likely to produce results (an exception may be with SSRIs). However, once this has been done and all classes have been tried, as well as augmentations and combinations, it may still be worthwhile to use other drugs from the same class when a drug has previously failed. Knowledge of drug effects remains incomplete, and trial-and-error efforts will at times be successful.

5. *Different approaches.* In cases where psychopharmacological treatments are ineffective or have limited effects, therapists should consider other options. These may include ECT, light therapy for those with seasonal changes, exercise regimens, or increased psychotherapeutic contact.

6. *Determination.* Therapists must understand the particularly debilitating and destructive nature of depression that is unresponsive to treatment. It places great demands on a therapist, both intellectually and

emotionally. Large reserves of courage, strength, and determination will need to be made available to a desperate patient.

As an extension of these considerations, consultation can be very helpful to a therapist. It can serve to focus a review of the course of treatment, to help the therapist maintain perspective, and to provide an appropriate outlet for ventilation and catharsis. Attending to the needs of the therapist is an ongoing issue for such treatment, but this should occur outside the immediate realm of the therapy.

MANAGEMENT OF SUICIDALITY

The risk of suicide among depressed patients is substantial: One of every 10 people with depression will die of suicide (Robins et al., 1959; Roy-Byrne et al., 1988). Moreover, almost all people with depression experience at least some passive suicidal ideation. The best protection against suicide is the effective treatment of the depression. Therefore, all that we have described about treating depression has been pertinent, if not crucial, to suicide prevention.

Suicidal crises among the depressed usually involve the convergence of several factors and their translation into the perception that life, as it is presently being experienced, is unbearable. The immediate affects experienced by a suicidal person may include anguish, helplessness, hopelessness, and/or anger. There is a sense that whatever is the source of such torture will be timeless and unremitting. From this perspective, suicide seems a reasonable solution. The elements that combine to create this state of mind include the following:

1. *The depression itself.* Depression, with its inherently painful affects, distorted cognition, dysfunctional regressive pull, and quality of timelessness, is a powerful force.

2. *Acute stressors.* Acute situations of disappointment, loss, rejection, or failure are intensified by the depression, and in turn worsen the feelings associated with the depression.

3. *Inadequate opposition.* There is an acute failure of those beliefs or relationships that oppose the depressive distortions and sustain perspective and hope. These include religious and philosophical beliefs that oppose suicide or make the person more fearful of the consequences of suicide than of the pain of living; those relationships (including the one with the therapist) that are allied with residual healthy perspectives, despite the depression and acute disruption; and those relationships with people who provide comfort, love, and meaning and who would suffer

more from the patient's suicide than they are deemed to suffer from the patient's depression. (There is an associated risk of homicide to protect loved ones [often a patient's children] from either the pain of the patient's suicide or the pain inherent in living, or alternately to protect them by "keeping them with" the patient).

These three factors may lead to a suicidal wish or even intent, which may become either an unsuccessful attempt or a completed suicide because of the fourth factor:

4. *Opportunity/ choice of method.* Lethality is determined more by the destructive potential of the instrument or method of suicide than the specific intent, although these are often consistent. Disparities in either direction (i.e., lethal intent and a nonlethal method, or vice versa) may result from ignorance, accidents, or ambivalence. A handful of benzodiazepine tablets may put one to sleep, whereas the same number of amitriptyline tablets may be lethal. Similarly, sliced wrists will probably clot, but a punctured abdominal aorta will not. A bullet can disable or kill. In short, the fact that a suicide attempt is unsuccessful does not define its motivation. The recognition of ambivalence does not reduce the seriousness of disturbance or warrant misattribution of motives, regardless of the burden placed upon the therapist. Having a residual innate will to live does not necessarily diminish the intensity of the wish to die; it may simply deflect the effort to die.

The tasks of the therapist treating a suicidal patient are to take each of these variables into account and counter them whenever possible.

With regard to the depression, the therapist should again focus on the manifestations of the depression as artifacts exerting great force and influence, but creating a distorted picture of the way things are. The therapist should also stress that most of these distortions are state-dependent and time-limited, and that they will change as the depression is treated. At the same time, there is an emphasis on whatever means are being used to treat the depression medically and on a repetitive, systematic examination of the patient's various options.

In dealing with an acute stressor, the therapist will find it useful to remind the patient (who will have forgotten) about the variety of coping skills the patient has employed in the past to solve or adjust to problems and crises paralleling the immediate stressful situation. The therapist can further demonstrate the variety of ways in which the issues exacerbated by this crisis interact with elements of depression to intensify the distorted perceptions that are pressing the patient toward suicide. Suicide should not be a "permanent solution to a temporary problem," as the advice columnist Ann Landers has put it. The therapist has already begun to build opposition to suicide by challenging and (ideally) undermining distorted perceptions and by describing various treatment options that will contribute to a sense of hope. When a patient has religious or moral objections to suicide, or relational ties to sustain him or her, these should certainly be examined with increasing elaboration, reinforcement, and support.

Perhaps the most crucial element here is the establishment of the safest possible "holding environment" that utilizes the therapeutic relationship. In the most extreme circumstances, or while there is sufficient uncertainty with insufficient protection, patients may need hospitalization, probably on a closed unit with continuous supervision. Two cautionary comments are pertinent here. First, therapists should never underestimate the seriousness of suicidal ideas, intentions, and attempts; these reflect deep pain, which can be deadly. Second, therapists should also never overestimate the power of religion, love, and therapeutic bonds; depression can override them. Even in cases where hospitalization may not be necessary, therapists should be aware that suicidal patients' emotional states may fluctuate greatly and that what looks like stability at one moment may quickly become instability or even unwavering lethal intent.

Patients whose intent is nonlethal but who nonetheless feel pressure toward suicide need access to their therapists. At periods of greater suicidal ideation or struggle, therapists should arrange to see their patients more frequently and/or arrange regular telephone contact. There should be a preestablished plan for what such a patient should do under threatening circumstances. This plan may include (1) having a prescribed set of coping skills to ward off or contend with suicidal feelings; (2) calling a friend or family member; (3) calling the therapist; (4) calling a suicide hotline; (5) going to an emergency room; (6) listening to a tape that the patient and therapist have prerecorded for such a time; and (7) other creative approaches. At times it will be useful to have a written contract, both to utilize the therapeutic relationship to underscore the patient's commitment to being safe, and to specify the steps for circumstances in which the patient may feel desperate, impulsive, and confused. Again, two caveats are in order. First, a therapist should not overestimate the value of a contract; there is no recourse to a breach of contract. Second, if the patient has agreed to forestall suicide and speak with the therapist, there must be a fail-safe method of contacting the therapist or a substitute.

Many patients will have experienced previous suicidal states. Therapists must search among these with their patients for opportunities to apply life-saving maneuvers to the current situation. It can be a powerful option to employ a patient's previous solutions to the same problem, whenever this is possible.

Having lived through such states with patients can also guide a therapist toward the intervention that will help to undermine a particular person's "moral imperative" to die. Among the more profound lessons that are likely to have been a part of both a therapist's and a patient's experience are that the patient has survived a prior suicidal state and that this state had the capacity to change. The therapist's conviction about this possibility may be more powerful than the patient's; if so, the therapist must convey it as convincingly as possible. When an antidepressant has been used successfully in the past to abort such a state, both parties have witnessed this change and can attest not only to the likelihood or possibility of its recurrence, but also to the state-dependent nature of the suicidal feelings. As a depressed physician said following the sudden disappearance of her suicidal preoccupation after the introduction of an SSRI, "Serotonin sure stops my suicidality." This statement reflects not simply the treatability of such a state, but its artifactual nature: In depression, suicidal states are not existentially but biologically driven.

The steps necessary to limit opportunities for suicide are usually carried out before a suicidal crisis occurs. Getting guns out of the home or into the temporary custody of a significant other should be done long before a crisis occurs, if possible. The choice of antidepressant should be determined mostly by efficacy, but is often made on the basis of safety. Many of the newer antidepressants have a much greater margin of safety than TCAs or MAOIs. In cases where a less safe drug is more effective, the margin of safety may be increased by dispensing the drug in small amounts.

Regardless of the specific maneuvers that are used to counter elements of the suicidal state, the most powerful force in guiding a patient through such a crisis will be the therapeutic alliance. The therapist must continually and repeatedly ally himself or herself with the patient and the patient's distress, while conveying a conviction of their capacity to get through the crisis together. The therapist may say things like this:

> "We have been through this before, and I know that you will feel different from the way you do now."
> "You have shown that you have the ability and strength to bear this a while longer, until you feel better."
> "This is the depression talking."
> "The things that seem overwhelming at this moment will be solvable when you are back to being yourself."

These are sustaining words, not platitudes, when delivered with compassion and conviction.

Conversely, conveying to a patient that a nonlethal overdose or other attempt was a "gesture," a "manipulation," or "histrionics" will undermine an alliance or potential for alliance and increase the patient's risk. Often these countertransference responses are part of a therapist's broader rationale for limiting involvement ("limit setting"), or even ways of punishing a patient for having the gall to express anguish or rage in a way that is upsetting to the therapist (Maltsberger & Buie, 1974). More appropriate responses, regardless of how the therapist may be reacting internally, include empathy for the primary state: "You must be in great pain to strike out in such a way."

·6·

Treatment Planning, Design, and Conduct

In Chapter 5, we have discussed the various elements of BIPD. We have described the recognition of depression's manifestations and of its impact on various aspects of personality functioning, as well as the development of strategies to limit these consequences. We have emphasized the primary biological underpinnings of clinical depression, despite the numerous possible psychological factors (developmental factors, dynamic issues, and present stressors), that may contribute to it. We have also emphasized the autonomous quality of depression once it has developed. Stressors may precipitate the depressed state or aggravate it once it is in progress; however, the depression itself becomes the primary driving force for many other changes.

Having defined techniques for treating depression, how do we organize these into a structure that can be offered to patients, taught to clinicians, and researched for its efficacy? How much of what do patients need? In order to help clinicians determine patient's specific therapeutic needs, we turn first in this chapter to issues of assessment.

ASSESSMENT

The following outline is a useful guide to the assessment of a depressed patient:

    Assessment of the depressioon
        Diagnosis
        Lifeline
        Profile

Assessment of functional risks
    Interpersonal risks
    Risks to job and role functions
    Risks to self and life
Assessment of the patient's assets and resources
    Developmental milestones, conflicts, and coping skills
    Support systems
    Motivational systems
Assessment of current stressors
Assessment of the patient's insight
Formulation or assessment summary

Assessment of the Depression

The first part of assessment deals not only with the specific diagnosis of depression, but also with the features that give the patient's depression its particular character, variability, and contours over time. A depressive episode that is part of a bipolar disorder will have implications for treatment that differ from those of dysthymic disorder, an episode of recurrent major depressive disorder, or a "double depression." The course of the depression over time will be somewhat predictive of its future course, especially when there has been a pattern of recurrent episodes with increasing frequency.

Beyond establishing a diagnosis, it is essential to obtain a lifetime picture of the course of depression in the patient. Whenever possible, this should be done by using both the patient's and other family members' recollections to construct a "lifeline" identifying previous episodes of depression (Post et al., 1988). For each episode, the time, the duration, and some relative measure of depth or intensity should be noted (see Figure 6.1). Also included in the lifeline should be brief notations concerning treatment (both psychopharmacological and psychotherapeutic) and significant life events and stressors. Setting down all these features of depression in this concrete fashion is helpful for both patient and therapist. In particular, the lifeline underscores for the patient the quality of depression as an "entity"—a view central to the BIPD approach.

In addition to using the lifeline to establish the "big picture," it is valuable to establish a profile of the salient features of the patient's depression. This should include the order in which features tend to be recruited as the depressed state appears and worsens, and, conversely, the order in which they leave as the state resolves. Although there can be marked changes in the symptomatic expression of depression from one episode to the next, or even within the time frame of a single episode, patients will usually be aware that some symptoms or other features seem

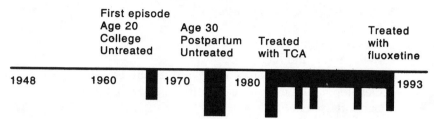

FIGURE 6.1. "Lifeline" chart of depression in a woman in her 40s with recurrent major depressive disorder and dysthymic disorder (see Case 3, Chapter 8).

to herald the return or exacerbation of their depression, and that others appear only when the depression becomes more severe. It is also important to note whether the features appear to evolve insidiously or to occur abruptly. A profile of depressive features usually reflects specific symptoms but may also highlight other elements of the language of depression, including personality or functional changes. The purpose of the profile is to establish "anchor points" to be used by patient and therapist for both identification and intervention at important points in the course of depression. For many patients, these serve as warning signals of the need to ask for help; for others, as a means of establishing perspective; and for still others, as indications for instituting changes in psychopharmacological treatment.

The establishment of a profile is particularly important for those patients whose depression appears insidiously and without their awareness. Being able to identify a particular outlook, behavior, or thought that raises their consciousness about the depression can be crucial for such patients. People are quite idiosyncratic in their anchor points, particularly in regard to which symptom or other feature is the first to appear. It may be trouble sleeping, a loss of enthusiasm, fatigue, or some other distinct symptom. Or it may be a tendency to be politically disgruntled, the appearance of wanderlust, or dissatisfaction with one's job. In cases where the onset of depression is heralded by philosophical or behavioral changes rather than symptoms, the risks of acting upon such state-dependent changes are greater than they are in cases where clear-cut symptoms permit patients to identify the return or worsening of their depression and to anticipate corresponding changes in outlook. Therefore, a profile can be especially informative and helpful for patients who do not experience clear "warning signs."

A profile of the depression, both historical and current, will also include the major target symptoms for psychopharmacological intervention—in other words, "core" symptoms of depression that are responsive to antidepressants. These can be assessed qualitatively or can be measured serially by using such widely available self-assessment tools as the Beck Depression Inventory (Beck et al., 1961) or the Zung Self-Rating Depression Scale (Zung, 1965). The reasons for following such target symptoms are to measure the effectiveness of intervention and to observe fluctuations in the severity of depression over time.

Finally, as noted above, the profile of depression should identify those symptoms or features that are "last to go" as depression resolves, or that may be residual features indicating an incomplete remission. Research (Kupfer et al., 1992; Keller et al., 1986) suggests the importance of achieving full remission—not only because of the advantages inherent in not being depressed, but also because the chances of relapse decrease when remission is complete. Therefore, establishing indices for this state is essential. At times, patients and therapists relax their efforts once initial pharmacological intervention has reduced symptoms by 50% or 75% or even 90%; however, aggressive management of depression should seek 100% remission of symptoms wherever possible.

Two sample profiles of depressive features are provided in Tables 6.1 and 6.2. Table 6.1 is the profile of a 50-year-old male executive with three episodes of depression within 3 years (see Case 2, Chapter 8); this profile is essentially symptom-driven. Table 6.2 is the profile of a professional woman in her early 30s with a 20-year history of depression (see Case 5, Chapter 8); her profile is marked by both philosophical changes and concrete symptoms.

Assessment of Functional Risks

In addition to the suffering that is a direct effect of depression's characteristic depressive mood changes, anxiety, anguish, and despair, clinicians must assess the potential risks to depressed patients in terms of their relationships, their work and role functions, and their suicidal potential. Accurate assessment of all these risks depends upon a clinician's and patient's ability to appreciate the full impact of depression in each of these areas. We have developed the San Diego Depressive Language Scales for patients' and therapists' use in identifying distress, dysfunction, and risk in the interpersonal, work-related, and intrapsychic domains. Appendix 6.1 presents these scales, which can and should be used for educational as well as assessment purposes. They are meant not only to identify potential elements of depression, but to initiate further exploration and therapeutic interventions concerning areas of risk to a depressed individual.

TABLE 6.1. Profile of Depressive Features in a 50-Year-Old Executive

Presenting features:	Diminished sleep
	Worry
	Short temper with family
	Realization that he is "not himself"
Target symptoms:	Sleep: 2–4 hours a night (vs. 7)
	Moderate fatigue
	Moderately lowered energy
	Marked irritability
	Minimal concentration
	Mildly decreased pleasure
	Absent libido
Residual symptoms:	Diminished libido

TABLE 6.2. Profile of Depressive Features in a Professional Woman in Her 30s

Presenting features:	Urge to change jobs and move
	Dissatisfaction with relationships
	Self-deprecation
Target symptoms:	Depressed mood
	Irritability
	Lowered energy
	Fatigue
	Appetite disturbance
	Pleasure only from close friend, dog
Residual symptoms:	Fatigue

Assessment of the Patient's Assets and Resources

Assessment of a depressed person should cover not only the depression itself and the risks associated with it, but also the strengths, capacities, skills, and supports the person has available for dealing with the depression and its impact on his or her life. This part of assessment includes the evaluation of the highest levels of adaptation the person has achieved developmentally, as well as the current levels. To the extent possible, these dimensions should be evaluated from a depression-free perspective; that is, the inquiry should be focused on points in time when the patient has not been affected by the depression, *and* it should be conducted when the patient (or significant other) can reflect upon such issues without the distortions introduced by a current state of depression.

Developmental Milestones, Conflicts, and Coping Skills

Have there been significant traumas, losses, or deaths, and if so, how has the patient coped with them? What have been the advantages and problems associated with various relationships—those with family members, friends, colleagues, teachers/supervisors, and romantic partners? What levels of accomplishment has the person achieved in his or her education and career? What areas of interest and pleasure has he or she pursued? Has depression impaired development in any of these areas? What are the patient's continuing sources of conflict? What are his or her major modes of coping? That is, does the patient tend to use intellectual, sublimatory, expressive, avoidant, or impulsive means of dealing with problems? And, to whatever extent this can be determined, what are the state-dependent differences between the patient's ego-adaptive coping strategies (ones that reflect optimal development) and his or her more regressive and depression-driven strategies?

Support Systems

What are the personal and institutional supports upon which the depressed person has relied? Who are the family members, friends, colleagues, associates, and authorities who provide warmth, pleasure, direction, and structure? What affiliations exist with church, schools, sporting or charitable organizations, and social clubs? Whom does the person call when he or she is in need?

Motivational Systems

What are the purposes, directions, and motives that have converged at the point of the patient's best level of functioning? How has he or she arrived at this point, and what are the defining characteristics of this point? This is not an assessment of unknown, unconscious motivations, but of the conscious forces that have driven, pushed, or seduced the person to develop a specific career, establish a family, and lead a particular kind of life. This is an assessment of the most optimistic vision to which the person may have subscribed, regardless of the condition of that vision at the moment; it may well be changed and distorted by current depression or by the impact of prior depression.

The assessment of the patient's accomplishments, strengths, assets, supports, and motivations should allow the therapist, in developing a treatment plan, to answer these questions: What strengths can be drawn from the patient? What supports are available from the outside? And what deficits exist that may need to be supplemented by the therapist? Quite importantly, this phase of assessment provides the therapist with a vision of what is possible without interference from the depression or its destructive effects.

Assessment of Current Stressors

Although there is generally an effort to identify current stressors as external environmental events that are affecting the patient and that may be contributing to the precipitation or aggravation of a depressive disorder, it is common to see a clinical picture in which there is limited interaction between the perceived stressor and the patient's depression, or even in which the depression may have caused the stressor. Examples of the latter occur when a patient's depression leads to loss of employment or the end of a marriage. We see the existence of an illness-driven stressor as no less a stressor and no less the focus of therapeutic attention.

Assessment of the Patient's Insight

Because of the centrality of education within the BIPD model, the determination of the patient's perception of his or her disorder is crucial. The easiest way to approach this issue is simply to ask, "What do you think is wrong with you?" There are three general categories of insight: (1) correct insight, (2) perplexity, and (3) incorrect insight.

Depressed patients with correct insight enter treatment with the recognition that there is something wrong and that whatever it may be has made them different persons. They are "not themselves." They know when they are "themselves," and they have a good appreciation and understanding of who they are at such times. They know that they are depressed and that when depressed they are "ill," although they may have little or no knowledge of the nature of the illness. Some of these patients may actually enter treatment with a very sophisticated scientific understanding of depression, as well as full comprehension of its symptomatic expression and its idiosyncratic effects on their thinking, functioning, regressive inclinations, and efforts to adapt in response to depression. Obviously, these are patients whose education will require less active intervention on the part of their therapists.

A second group of patients will come for evaluation without a clue as to what is wrong. They may say that they are depressed because they feel bad, but they are unlikely to define themselves as *having* depression: Their depressive affect may seem only a small part of a myriad of distressing affects, disrupted functions, and deteriorating circumstances that leave them confused, frightened, and overwhelmed. Upon inquiry, they have no preconceived notions of what is wrong, but are likely to be highly receptive to and appreciative of any information their clinicians can give them. They need education and are quite ready for it.

The third group of patients have a great deal of insight, but it is *wrong*—because of the distortions created by the depression, misconceptions about the nature of the disorder, or both. Patients who make errors of distortion may realize that they are depressed, but are sufficiently "captive" that they are convinced about the validity of their negative perceptions of themselves (their fundamental inadequacy, lack of commitment, excessive dependency, nihilism, etc.). Patients who make errors of misattribution may have a full recognition of their depression, but interpret it incorrectly as a reflection of an unhappy home life, Oedipal conflicts, or poor self-esteem—all manifestations of being "screwed up."

Patients with depressive distortions will need specific education focused on the language of depression—a task made more difficult in this group, because of the already manifest predisposition to be "captured." Those patients with misattributions will require reeducation, which often requires considerable proactivity on the part of therapists: anticipating the personal and cultural transmission of strong beliefs that reflect obsessional and narcissistic needs for control and mastery; tracing the evolution of such beliefs; and demonstrating their fallaciousness with the aid of scientific data on the biology of depression.

Formulation or Assessment Summary

Once the clinician has completed his or her assessments of the patient's depression, functional risks, assets and resources, current stressors, and insights about his or her illness, it is important to develop a formulation that integrates all of these levels of understanding. This formulation becomes the clinician's initial working guide to treatment planning in all spheres of a biopsychosocial approach.

This summary should be presented to the patient with as much depth and complexity as he or she can comprehend. Feedback from the patient is invited and clarifications by the clinician are desirable. Both clinician and patient should understand that this formulation may change over time, and is only a "work in progress." (See Chapter 8 for examples.)

STRUCTURE OF TREATMENT SESSIONS

The structure of sessions in BIPD follows from the specific tasks pursued by the therapist and patient. Although the order of these tasks may proceed from the patient's perceived area of greatest difficulty (driven by discomfort), each session should include the following:

1. Review of the status of depression
2. Evaluation of psychopharmacological treatment
3. Review of progress in coping skills
4. Examination of current life stressors

A fifth task, consultation with significant others, should be included whenever it is necessary or desirable (see below).

Review of the Status of Depression

The therapist should *always* review the current status of the patient's depression—the specific symptoms, their frequency and intensity, and the extent to which they are improving or changing in response to treatment. Emphasis throughout should be on the patient's broadening consciousness of the elements of depression as he or she experiences these.

As part of this expansion of the patient's awareness, there should be a continuing reassessment of the language of depression as it manifests itself in work-related, interpersonal, and self-conceptual domains. Wherever there is an indication that the patient is perceiving depressive features as existential truths, the therapist should challenge these perceptions. How much time is spent in therapeutic sessions reviewing such issues depends on the degree of turmoil and risk they may create, as well as on the patient's capacity to recognize them and retain perspective about them.

Assessment of suicide risk should be part of every session. For those patients who are struggling with suicidal ideas, impulses, wishes, and plans, this may be the central focus of therapeutic sessions. For those in whom suicidal preoccupation or risk is low, there need be only passing attention. However, the systematic inclusion of some level of risk assessment reflects the recognition of suicide as an ever-present concern in working with depressed patients.

Evaluation of Psychopharmacological Treatment

The therapist should also spend part of each session evaluating the patient's compliance with psychopharmacological treatment. This should include evaluation of problems with the treatment—either psychological problems or physical side effects. Physicians will be assessing the latter for the purpose of making appropriate adjustments in dosage. Non-physicians will attend to psychological management of resistance and will make medical referrals when these are appropriate. Because many patients struggle with the issue of taking medication, it should not surprise therapists of any discipline that even a minor medical complication is likely to escalate such resistance. Although nonphysician psychotherapists may be correctly reluctant to give medical advice, it is important that they attend to potential disruptions in psychopharmacological treatment—not only by encouraging close follow-up with prescribing psychiatrists or other physicians, but also by examining and helping patients to understand other factors in their resistance.

Review of Progress in Coping Skills

Each session should likewise include a review of progress in the patient's use of more adaptive cognitive and behavioral coping skills. Every patient will have a different set of depressive responses that will require modification. How effective are patients in modifying their depressed mood by examining and challenging their negative perceptions or by engaging in one or another behavior? When depression is unshakable, how well can patients insulate themselves from suffering its effects? How can they struggle to avoid further deterioration? Therapists and patients must regularly examine the tools that the patients are employing to cope with these situations. We have used the exercises in Appendix 6.2 to help patients review some of their available means of coping with depression.

Examination of Current Life Stressors

Central to an examination of current life stressors is the awareness of the potential contribution of depression to the perception of such stressors. Even where there are clearly definable and independent stressful events occurring in the context of depression, the therapist and patient should be mindful of the depressive inclination to intensify the impact of these events, whether interpersonal, financial, health-related, or of some other type.

Current stressors may lead to exploration of areas of conflict that are unrelated to depression. Long-standing dynamic themes may be examined productively. Such directions are safer to take once a patient's depression is under some control and the state-dependent regressions are less likely to drive and distort such explorations. During the throes of acute depression, for example, an exploration of the patient's relationship to his or her supervisor at work will probably intensify dynamic themes of inadequacy and overcontrol, while excluding perceptions of positive affiliation or productive competitiveness. Thus, the timing of such exploration in the course of psychotherapy is important.

Consultation with Significant Others

Consultation with significant others is likely to be task-specific and dependent on the state of treatment. It is desirable, at a minimum, that a spouse or family member be included during the initial assessment and at some critical points in treatment, as described in Chapter 5. When significant others are present, the treatment session is likely to change in emphasis, although all of the first four tasks described above should also be included.

Although each session should include some focus on (1) the current state of depression, (2) psychopharmacological treatment, (3) utilization of coping skills, and (4) current life stressors, the present discussion is not meant to restrict the scope of psychotherapeutic work. The skilled therapist may find other specific areas of application. However, the same caveat applies here as elsewhere: The therapist must be sure that the material to be explored is not a directly significant and/or distorted product of the depression itself.

LENGTH AND FREQUENCY OF TREATMENT SESSIONS

The length and frequency of treatment sessions have always represented a compromise between the practical and financial needs of therapists and the emotional needs and financial resources of patients. Because financial considerations are increasingly determined by third-party payers in the private or public sector, this issue has become less a point of direct negotiation between therapists and patients, and this trend is likely to continue with the development of national health care policy in the United States. Traditionally, where psychotherapy has been concerned, there has been a general view of "more is better," especially when the assumptions about the nature of psychopathology have been "what you don't know can hurt you" and "you can never know enough."

The guideline for the length and frequency of BIPD sessions is "as little as necessary and as much as necessary." Behind this view are a number of principles operating to press for both more and less intensive and extensive treatment. In a general sense, we anticipate that long-term treatment is going to be a necessity for the majority of patients who have either a continual struggle with depression or frequently recurring episodes. It is the exceptional patient who has a single episode that resolves without recurrence, and even in those instances where this proves to be the case, there is no way to know at the time of the index episode what the future will bring. So, even in cases where there will be no recurrence, the patients may live with the specter of recurrence and may need to plan to deal with it.

The most powerful issue determining the "as little as necessary" side of the equation is the chronicity-driven struggle for autonomy that almost all depressed patients face. The illness itself represents the greatest threat to personal autonomy, as it undermines daily functioning, careers, relationships, and self-esteem. A further consequence of chronicity is that ongoing or intermittent treatment with a therapist will foster the development of dependency upon the therapist. This is both inevitable and desirable as a vehicle for helping a patient improve the quality of his or her life. However, this dependency also has the potential for further undermining the self-esteem and functional capacities of a patient who comes to rely too much upon the therapist. In analytic therapies, the intensifying regressive quality of dependency is a desirable development in the evolution of a transference neurosis to be studied. In BIPD, by contrast, dependency is a necessary and ubiquitous feature that must be limited and balanced, and whose excess is detrimental. Aside from psychopharmacological management, all of the techniques utilized in BIPD are such that patients can and should learn to incorporate them into their daily lives. (There are also many patients who become extraordinarily sophisticated about psychopharmacology, and many who, regardless of their level of knowledge, participate actively in decision making.)

On the other side of the equation are those forces that call for more treatment, more often. These include the following:

1. *Severity of the episode.* A severe depressive episode obviously requires more intense monitoring and more active support, especially when there are immediate risks to work, hazards to relationships, or suicidal struggles.

2. *Early phases of treatment.* In the beginning, a patient requires more education about depression and exposure to methods of exploring, understanding, and coping with the manifestations of depression.

3. *A lack of social support.* Of course, over time, one of the goals of therapy should be the elaboration of the patient's social support system.

4. *The inclination of the patient to be "captured" by depression.* Although a major focus of treatment is on the development of a patient's capacity to maintain perspective, there are those patients whose depressions always seem to override these efforts, leaving them continually vulnerable and necessitating more contact with their therapists.

5. *The absence of monitors.* In cases where there are no people who can serve the functions of giving patients feedback about their depres-

sion and lending them perspective, these tasks are more likely to fall upon therapists.

6. *The absence of a treatment alliance.* An essential element of a treatment alliance is the patient's trust that the therapist will be available and will help the patient to obtain what he or she needs—not too little or too much—when it is needed. Once that trust has developed (as in the rapprochement phase of childhood development), the patient will have sufficient confidence to struggle with the depression as best he or she can, and to turn to the therapist in time of need.

The duration and frequency of treatment sessions should be based on the individual patient's need and should always be adjustable. The guidelines we have developed through years of practice and struggle reflect a general theme with variations: more frequently early in treatment, and a gradually diminishing frequency with time. This translates into the following approximate schedule for a presenting episode of depression: psychotherapy weekly for 2 months, biweekly for 2 months, and monthly thereafter. Sessions usually last between 45 and 60 minutes, especially at the beginning of treatment, and may continue indefinitely in that time frame or may be shortened to 30 minutes. The factors listed above will determine length of sessions as well as frequency, both at the time of a given episode and as treatment continues over time.

In addition to face-to-face sessions, the use of the telephone can be an important adjunct to treatment. It may be essential for a suicidal patient: Being able to talk with the therapist, or with some other professional in circumstances where the therapist is not always available, may literally be life-saving. However, there are other ways in which telephone contact can be quite helpful without fostering excessive dependency. A well-timed, brief phone contact may lend perspective at a time when the patient may have lost his or hers and is at risk of compromising a relationship or job or is simply feeling overwhelmed. For a psychiatrist, a few minutes' consultation may reassure a patient about a side effect and keep him or her from discontinuing necessary medication. Similarly, a brief phone discussion of a crisis or change in the state of the depression, instead of coming to the office for a session, may enhance the patient's self-esteem.

As treatment continues beyond the early phases and proceeds over time, necessitated by continuing (though, one hopes, diminishes) manifestations of depression, the amount of contact can become quite minimal. This may be especially true for those patients who have developed a good treatment alliance; are well educated about their depression; are in good control of their symptoms; have good internal resources and good support systems; and are able to maintain perspective even with episodic fluctuations in mood. Such patients can be seen with diminishing frequency or even on an "as needed" basis determined by themselves. In cases where antidepressant medications are being prescribed, the same principles may determine the frequency of contact, though many psychiatrists (and other prescribing physicians) may have personally determined limits to how frequently they feel they need to see patients. As a result, some patients may be seen as little as once or twice a year, with occasional supplementary phone calls to maintain contact, while remaining in "active" treatment. At times, such variations will be determined by therapists' comfort as much as or more than by patients' need. The therapeutic alliance is often the most critical factor in allowing such limited contact. However, just as some forms of parental "benign neglect" confirm the capabilities and autonomy of their children, therapists' hovering in the background and being available can convey a powerful message of confidence to patients struggling with a potentially devastating chronic illness.

CONDUCT OF THE PSYCHOTHERAPIST

The treatment of depression should be an active process, and the therapist should be not only active (as all therapists claim to be, insofar as they all claim to be thinking about what their patients are saying all the time) but interactive. The primary goal of the therapist is to help the patient fight depression, and the behavior of the therapist should reflect his or her participation in this battle. This work involves a good deal of inquiry, probing, and empathizing, as well as confronting, explaining, directing, and supporting.

BIPD is not a process of guided self-exploration on the part of the patient, in which free association will lead to self-understanding. On the contrary, free association driven by depression will lead to a ever-widening abyss of distortion, self-recrimination, and despair if the patient is left to his or her own devices. Traditional, regressive therapies can be quite destructive for depressed patients and are contraindicated for those who are actively suicidal. Such treatment only increases distortion, confusion, and regression. Depressed patients need therapists who will provide structure, help them direct and correct their thinking, and actively support the strengths that they themselves cannot perceive or utilize.

The verbal interaction is largely conversational, and considerable creativity and flexibility are required of the therapist. Despite the fact that there is a general structure to the therapeutic sessions, the therapist should have a facility in moving among various stances: empathic listening to the misery within a patient's existence; confrontational arguments with the patient over the distortions that the depression creates; persistent advice giving in order to prevent the patient from acting upon an "existential" issue; and cheerleading on behalf of a more optimistic outcome than the patient is able to perceive.

There are difficulties facing therapists who use BIPD as their approach to treating depressed patients. The type of treatment we are describing in this book is likely to be described as "supportive psychotherapy," which, of course, all good psychotherapies are. The problem with such a label is that it has traditionally defined what a psychotherapy is not, rather than what it is. Nonpsychoanalytic therapists have traditionally struggled with the idea that they are providing the "brass" of other psychotherapies rather than the "gold" of psychoanalysis, and that they are helping people cope rather than "changing structure." Furthermore, techniques of various supportive psychotherapies have been devalued because they appeal to common sense and can be understood and learned by anyone, in contrast to analytic psychotherapy, which for many is less comprehensible and can only be learned under highly prescribed circumstances. These factors have contributed to the overvaluation of psychoanalysis—an overvaluation that persists, despite a lack of scientific validity. Still, because of the appealing intellectual heritage of the psychoanalytic movement, these themes continue to make some therapists reluctant to pursue less valued psychotherapeutic avenues.

Therapists' difficulties in treating depressed patients are primarily the consequences of the disorder itself. Empathic work with depressed patients can "rub off" onto therapists, regardless of their capacity to maintain necessary clinical objectivity. The devastation that depression visits upon patients can become a burden for therapists, as well as coloring their mood at least temporarily—and over time with increasing investment—in ways that can be disturbing and persistent. From a therapeutic standpoint, therapists can use these experiences as a means both of monitoring their patients' state of mind, and of mobilizing the patients as well as themselves to perceive this state and either utilize it productively or defend against it reasonably.

It is important that therapists not succumb to their patients' state of mind, for the sake of both therapists and patients. For this reason, therapists must be familiar with their own propensities toward depressive states and must develop the same capacity for maintaining insight and perspective that they teach to their patients. Therapists who themselves become "captives" of depressive states can prove quite detrimental to their patients. Such regressions can create depressive *folies à deux* in which depressive artifacts are reinforced and become "real," and no one is available to steer the patients back onto the right track.

Aside from therapists' abilities to manage their own depressive regressions, it is important that therapists of depressed patients have a general inclination toward optimism and a positive view of other people in which they readily perceive the others' strengths and virtues. Therapists who are cynical about life, critical of people, and oriented toward seeing pathology are not what the depressed need. Patients are already struggling with the force of their depression, and emphasizing what is wrong with themselves and the world. Incorporating cynical and critical therapist attitudes will be harmful. Positive attitudes are not things that can be feigned. Therapists cannot "act" appreciative and positive; they need to *be* so. An essential therapeutic process is a therapist's consistency in reflecting a patient's healthiest elements to balance the impact of depression. This should be reflected in both the therapist's states (see above) and traits.

In the face of continuing, refractory depression, even the most optimistic and capable therapists will experience feelings of frustration, helplessness, and at least transient despair. What is most crucial in such circumstances is to recognize that the culprit remains the depression, despite the fact that both patients and therapists often feel a sense of failure, self-recrimination, and pessimism. When patients become aware of this process in their therapists (and patients are often highly vigilant about the effects that their depression is having upon their therapists), they will become more upset in anticipation of the therapists' anger and blame toward them, and will fear being rejected or abandoned.

When a therapist in this situation is confronted by the patient's partially correct observation that the therapist is frustrated and may be angry or blaming, it is correct to acknowledge the struggle, but crucial to point out the broader reality. An example of a therapeutic response might be this: "It's been hard for me to see you suffering so much for so long, and frustrating to see that our best efforts have such limited effects. Depression can really be a monster—let's figure out what else we can do." Such a statement demonstrates that the therapist is struggling; that depression, and not the patient, is the culprit; that therapist and patient remain allied; and that their efforts will continue (i.e., it's not time to give up).

TRANSFERENCE AND COUNTERTRANSFERENCE ISSUES

BIPD is conducted in a planned and reinforced positive transference. Effective treatment relies on the maintenance of this positive transference. The therapist is seen as a benign, thoughtful, helpful, caring, giving person who has expertise, and in regard to the therapist–patient relationship, this should be true. Although the inherent limits of psychotherapy and the ethical restraint of the therapist may be frustrating to some patients, all but the most personality-disturbed will be able to tolerate and thrive in this situation. Because the treatment situation is highly structured and focused, there is less likelihood of developing intense transference reactions in BIPD than in more regressive forms of psychotherapy.

Although it is not the purpose of BIPD to study the evolution of highly idealized, dependent, erotic, or hostile transference material, it is essential that therapists recognize it when it appears and "manage" it. Management may involve "normalization" through matter-of-fact acknowledgment of the phenomenon, comments on how reasonable such feelings may be under these circumstances, and questions about whether a patient feels comfortable working with a therapist under the circumstances. Consider this example:

> A young depressed woman told her therapist that she found him very attractive, was having fantasies of sleeping with him, and thought he might agree. The therapist replied: "It's understandable, working so closely, and given your reliance on me and appreciation for my help, that such feelings would occur. Of course, it isn't possible. I hope your feelings won't keep us from being able to work together."

In other circumstances, some efforts to interpret (or at least partially interpret) transference reactions are well in keeping with the overall strategy of this treatment:

> A woman in treatment for many years became angry at her therapist for being uncaring and insensitive to her needs when he seemed distant to her at the time of a phone call. The therapist acknowledged that for him, the telephone did create something of a barrier to his empathy; however, he tried to reassure her of his concern. He went on to point out that the patient's response to him seemed very similar to feelings she had frequently experienced in relation to both her mother and her ex-husband, especially when she was depressed and feeling a heightened sense of vulnerability. This observation was used to examine the anger generated by her perceived dependency.

When transference material appears in such a way that it needs to be confronted, transference interpretations should be "made out of" the treatment situation whenever possible, rather than "read into" it. That is, the therapist should attempt to avoid intensifying the patient's transference by focusing on it or encouraging elaboration of it, as a therapist might in trying to develop a transference neurosis in an analytic psychotherapy. Finally, to limit patients' dependency on and idealization of their therapists, patients should be encouraged to work on their own within the treatment and to control their comings and goings in terms of the frequency of treatment once they have developed some mastery of the treatment techniques.

Countertransference difficulties usually occur in response to the intensification of hostile dependency. This, in turn, is an almost inevitable product of persistent depression and the failure of treatment efforts. As stated earlier, it is critical that a therapist and patient understand this as a normal product of "the enemy," lest they take it out on each other. At times, it is important that the patient be able to utilize the therapist as a repository for frustration, helplessness, and rage. This is certainly preferable to having the patient turn these emotions inward. Ideally, though, the therapist and patient will ally themselves and use this energy to fight the real culprit—the disease.

APPENDIX 6.1. SAN DIEGO DEPRESSIVE LANGUAGE SCALES

These exercises consist of groups of statements. For each item, read each statement carefully, then pick out the one statement that best describes how you have been feeling or acting during the past week including today. Circle the number of the statement you picked. If more than one statement in the group applies equally well, circle each one. Be sure to read each statement carefully.

Ranking the Effects of Depression on Your Interpersonal Relationships

1. 0 I get pleasure and satisfaction from my relationships.
   1 Occasionally I don't get pleasure or satisfaction from my relationships.
   2 I get no pleasure or satisfaction from my relationships.
   3 My relationships are unsatisfying and painful.

2. 0 I feel positive and respond to life.
   1 Occasionally I feel empty and unresponsive.
   2 I feel empty and unresponsive most of the time.
   3 I lack all feeling or feel "numb."

3. 0 I am flexible and resilient.
   1 I am less flexible and resilient than I used to be.
   2 I lack flexibility and resilience.
   3 I am rigid and unable to rebound from life's hardships.

4. 0 I enjoy being with other people and social situations.
   1 I sometimes avoid other people and social situations.
   2 I withdraw from other people and prefer to isolate myself from social situations.
   3 I dislike people and refuse to be in social situations.

5. 0 I look forward to and enjoy sex.
   1 Occasionally I don't enjoy sex.

    2   I don't enjoy sex most of the time.

    3   I avoid and dislike sex.

6.   0   I have a good sense of humor.

    1   Sometimes my sense of humor is poor.

    2   I have lost my sense of humor.

    3   I am a humorless and negative person.

7.   0   I am an independent and self-reliant person.

    1   I am less independent and self-reliant than I used to be.

    2   I feel needy and dependent on others.

    3   I cling to others and can't make it on my own.

8.   0   I appreciate other people who are trying to help me.

    1   I sometimes resent people who are trying to help me.

    2   I often resent people who are trying to help me.

    3   I resent and actively dislike people who are trying to help me.

9.   0   I am positive and hopeful.

    1   I am occasionally irritable, bitter, and cynical.

    2   I am often irritable, bitter, and cynical.

    3   I am pessimistic, bitter, and cynical most of the time.

10.   0   I am considerate and empathic toward myself and others.

    1   I sometimes lack consideration and empathy toward myself and others.

    2   I often lack consideration and empathy toward myself and others.

    3   I lack consideration and empathy toward myself and others most or all of the time.

11.   0   I can trust and rely on my relationships.

    1   Sometimes I feel like I can't trust or rely on my relationships.

    2   I feel more likely to lose or end relationships.

    3   I want to end relationships.

12.   0   I never have violent thoughts toward others.

    1   I occasionally have violent thoughts toward others.

    2   I often have violent thoughts toward others.

    3   I have recently acted on my violent thoughts and feelings.

13.   0   I am accepting and open-minded about those who are close to me.

    1   Sometimes I am unaccepting and critical about those who are close to me.

    2   I am often unaccepting and critical about those who are close to me.

    3   I am always unaccepting and critical about those who are close to me.

14.   0   I appreciate constructive criticism.

    1   I sometimes feel criticized and rejected.

    2   I often feel criticized or rejected.

    3   I frequently search for evidence that others are criticizing or rejecting me.

15.   0   I enjoy time by myself.

    1   Time by myself is not enjoyable.

2   I feel uncomfortable when I am by myself.
3   I feel isolated and desperately alone most of the time.

Ranking the Effects of Depression on Your Productive Capacities

16.   0   I wake up in the morning feeling rested.
      1   I occasionally have trouble sleeping.
      2   I wake up while I am sleeping and have trouble falling back to sleep.
      3   I wake up while I am sleeping and can't fall back to sleep.

17.   0   I have adequate physical and mental energy.
      1   I am sometimes physically and/or mentally tired.
      2   I am often physically and/or mentally tired.
      3   I am too tired to do anything.

18.   0   I enjoy how I spend my time.
      1   Sometimes I don't enjoy how I spend my time.
      2   I get little satisfaction from how I spend my time.
      3   Everything I do is a waste of time.

19.   0   I enjoy my day-to-day accomplishments.
      1   Sometimes I don't enjoy my day-to-day accomplishments.
      2   I belittle what I do accomplish because it has little value.
      3   Nothing that I do has any value.

20.   0   I feel self-confident.
      1   I sometimes lack self-confidence in my abilities.
      2   I lack self-confidence in my abilities.
      3   I have no self-confidence in my abilities.

21.   0   I can complete most tasks easily.
      1   I sometimes have trouble completing tasks.
      2   I often have trouble completing tasks.
      3   I am unable to complete any task.

22.   0   I can concentrate and focus on details.
      1   I sometimes have trouble concentrating and focusing on details.
      2   I often have trouble concentrating and focusing on details.
      3   I am unable to concentrate or focus on details.

23.   0   I enjoy being with others.
      1   I sometimes avoid being with others.
      2   I often avoid being with others.
      3   I am unable to spend time with others.

24.   0   I feel secure in my role at work.
      1   I sometimes worry that I may leave or lose my job.
      2   It is likely that I will leave or lose my job.
      3   I am about to or have already left/lost my job because of my state of mind.

25.   0   I get along well with my coworkers.
      1   I sometimes have trouble getting along with my coworkers.

2 I often have trouble getting along with my coworkers.

3 I am unable to get along with my coworkers.

26. 0 I make decisions easily.

1 I sometimes have trouble making decisions.

2 I often have trouble making decisions.

3 I am unable to make any decisions.

27. 0 I am irritated only occasionally and for "good reason."

1 I become irritated more often than I used to do.

2 I am frequently irritated.

3 I "blow up" in anger regularly.

28. 0 I am a patient person.

1 I am sometimes impatient.

2 I am frequently impatient.

3 I am impatient most or all of the time.

29. 0 I am a flexible person.

1 I am sometimes inflexible.

2 I am frequently inflexible.

3 I am inflexible and rigid most or all of the time.

30. 0 I enjoy my work and my life.

1 Sometimes I don't enjoy my work and my life.

2 I sometimes feel "burnt out."

3 I feel "burnt out" most or all of the time.

Ranking the Effects of Depression on Your Sense of Self

31. 0 I am interested in many things.

1 I don't have interest in things the way I used to.

2 I feel little interest in anything now.

3 Nothing will ever interest me again.

32. 0 I am self-reliant and can take care of myself.

1 I sometimes feel helpless.

2 I frequently feel helpless.

3 I am totally helpless.

33. 0 I rarely feel guilty.

1 I sometimes feel guilty.

2 I often feel guilty.

3 I am consumed with feelings of guilt and remorse.

34. 0 I feel like an adequate and worthwhile person.

1 I occasionally feel inadequate and unimportant.

2 I often feel inadequate and unimportant.

3 I feel inadequate and unimportant most or all of the time.

35. 0 I rarely feel confused.

1 I sometimes feel confused.

2 I often feel confused.

3 I feel confused most or all of the time.

36. 0 I feel loved and connected to others.
    1 Sometimes I don't feel loved or connected to others.
    2 I often feel unloved and isolated.
    3 I am unloved and isolated from others.

37. 0 I feel complete.
    1 I sometimes feel empty.
    2 I often feel empty.
    3 I feel empty most or all of the time.

38. 0 I feel hopeful most of the time.
    1 I feel less hopeful than I used to feel.
    2 I often feel hopeless.
    3 I feel hopeless most or all of the time.

39. 0 I feel attractive most of the time.
    1 I feel sometimes unattractive and unappealing.
    2 I often feel unattractive and unappealing.
    3 I feel unattractive and unappealing most of the time.

40. 0 I am an independent person.
    1 I sometimes feel dependent.
    2 I often feel dependent.
    3 I feel dependent most or all of the time.

41. 0 I am an optimistic person.
    1 I am less optimistic than I used to be.
    2 I am often pessimistic.
    3 I am pessimistic most or all of the time.

42. 0 I am usually successful in my role at work.
    1 I am rarely successful in my role at work.
    2 I am often a failure in my role at work.
    3 I am a complete failure in my role at work.

43. 0 I am usually successful at my role(s) as a parent, child, spouse, significant other, etc.
    1 I am rarely successful at my role(s) as a parent, child, spouse, significant other, etc.
    2 I am often a failure at my role(s) as a parent, child, spouse, significant other, etc.
    3 I am a complete failure at my role(s) as a parent, child, spouse, significant other, etc.

44. 0 I am satisfied with who I am now.
    1 I am not as satisfied with who I am as I used to be.
    2 I am usually unsatisfied with who I am and need to change.
    3 I need to make major changes in who I am.

45. 0 I am glad I am alive.
    1 Life is less important to me than it used to be.

2   I sometimes wish my life were shorter.
3   I wish I were dead.

Scoring

Add up your score for each of the three areas. If you circled more than one statement for a given item number, add the higher score. For example, for item number 41, if you circled both 1 (I am less optimistic than I used to be) and 3 (I am pessimistic most or all of the time), you should use 3, the higher score. Refer to the guidelines below to see how your depression is affecting the various areas of your life.

Interpersonal relationships:	1–15	Mild impact
	16–30	Moderate impact
	31+	Severe impact
Productive capacities:	1–15	Mild impact
	16–30	Moderate impact
	31+	Severe impact
Sense of self:	1–15	Mild impact
	16–30	Moderate impact
	31+	Severe impact

APPENDIX 6.2. COPING SKILLS EXERCISES

Below are a number of coping techniques that you may have used in the past or are using currently. Read each statement carefully, then circle how helpful this form of coping is for you.

Education as a Form of Coping

	Doesn't help			Helps a lot
1. I try to learn as much as I can about the problem.	0	1	2	3
2. I make a list of what I need to do.	0	1	2	3
3. I learn how other people coped with the same difficulty.	0	1	2	3
4. I draw on my past experiences.	0	1	2	3
5. I think about how a person I admire would handle the situation and use this as a model.	0	1	2	3
6. I ask a relative or friend I respect for advice.	0	1	2	3
7. I go over in my mind what I will say or do.	0	1	2	3

8.	I remember that the problem is separate from who I am as a person.	0	1	2	3

Modification of Pain/Overriding Mood as a Form of Coping

1.	I listen to a relaxation tape.	0	1	2	3
2.	I meditate or pray.	0	1	2	3
3.	I turn to work or other activities to take my mind off things.	0	1	2	3
4.	I daydream or imagine a better time or place than the one I am in now.	0	1	2	3
5.	I watch TV, listen to music, or rent a video.	0	1	2	3
6.	I take a bath.	0	1	2	3
7.	I exercise strenuously.	0	1	2	3
8.	I organize things (pay bills, clean closets, etc.).	0	1	2	3
9.	I spend time with a relative or friend.	0	1	2	3
10.	I read (a book, the newspaper, poems, etc.).	0	1	2	3
11.	I do crossword puzzles.	0	1	2	3
12.	I do something with my hands (sew, knit, carpentry, etc.).	0	1	2	3
13.	I do something creative (music, painting, pottery, etc.).	0	1	2	3
14.	I spend time outside (in the garden, at the beach, hiking, etc.) .	0	1	2	3

Transcending Distortion as a Form of Coping

1.	I feel that time will make a difference; the only thing to do is wait.	0	1	2	3
2.	I look for the silver lining; try to look on the bright side of things.	0	1	2	3
3.	I try not to act too hastily or follow my first hunch.	0	1	2	3
4.	I don't let it get to me; refuse to think about it too much.	0	1	2	3
5.	I try to keep my feelings from interfering with other things too much.	0	1	2	3
6.	I try to see things from another point of view.	0	1	2	3
7.	I remind myself about positive things in my life.	0	1	2	3

Enhancing Healthy Behavior
as a Form of Coping

1. I try to keep my schedule and routines the same.	0	1	2	3
2. I try to keep a regular sleep routine.	0	1	2	3
3. I drink three or fewer caffeinated drinks per day (coffee, tea, soda).	0	1	2	3
4. I drink one or fewer alcoholic drinks per day.	0	1	2	3
5. I smoke half a pack of cigarettes or less.	0	1	2	3
6. I eliminate extra stress from my life.	0	1	2	3
7. I try to eat balanced meals.	0	1	2	3
8. I try to distance myself from people who are abusive.	0	1	2	3

Scoring

Add up your scores for each of the four areas. Refer to the guidelines below to see how well various forms of coping work for you.

Education: Score >8 indicates this is a helpful form of coping for you.

Modification of pain-overriding mood: Score >14 indicates this is a helpful form of coping for you.

Transcending distortion: Score >7 indicates this is a helpful form of coping for you.

Eliminating maladaptive behavior: Score >8 indicates this is a helpful form of coping for you.

·7·

Comparison with Other Psychotherapies for Depression

To our knowledge, BIPD is the first form of psychotherapy for depression to be systematically based on the assumption that depression is at its core a biological disorder. Several other forms of psychotherapy, many of which have been codified in manuals and are taught and practiced in this standardized form, have been studied and used in conjunction with antidepressant medications. Karasu (1977, 1990) has described and compared these treatments, which include forms of short-term dynamically oriented psychotherapy (STDP), cognitive-behavioral therapy (CBT), and interpersonal psychotherapy (IPT). We have extended Karasu's descriptions and format to include BIPD in such comparisons. These psychotherapies differ from BIPD and from one another in terms of the following:

1. Theoretical conceptions of depressive pathology and etiology
2. Goals and implementation of psychotherapy
3. Psychotherapeutic techniques and practices
4. The patient–therapist relationship
5. Limitations and potentially harmful effects

In this chapter, we compare BIPD with STDP and other dynamic therapies, with CBT, and with IPT along these dimensions.

THEORETICAL CONCEPTIONS OF DEPRESSIVE PATHOLOGY AND ETIOLOGY

Psychodynamic theories of depressive pathology and etiology have evolved over the past century. They view depression as an ego regression—focused variably on a blockade of libido and unresolved oral conflict (Abraham 1911/1948), ambivalence over object loss with retroflexed anger (Freud, 1917/1955), or early narcissistic injury (Rado, 1927)—or as a fundamental ego state (Bibring, 1953). These theories have been discussed in greater detail in Chapter 2.

Cognitive theories of depression (e.g., Beck, 1976; Beck et al., 1979) emphasize personality-based and developmentally based distortions of thinking as the central pathological elements. Depression is viewed as driven by this distorted thinking about the self, the world, and the future. Behaviors based on these false beliefs are thought to feed into a negatively reinforcing cycle of evolving depression.

Interpersonal theories of depression (e.g., Klerman et al., 1984) postulate that although it is a multifactorial illness, the central forces contributing to depression are the patients' inadequate or unsatisfactory social relationships. These are thought to result from early losses, limited social skills, and/or maladaptive relatedness.

Biological theories suggest that the core of depressive pathology consists of altered chemical and neurophysiological processes, which are manifested in emotional, cognitive, and somatic interpersonal alterations. Depressive illness arises out of genetic vulnerability and nonspecific "stressors," which may be biological or psychological; however, the illness is an autonomous process that is independent of its precipitants or other predisposing factors. We have described these theories in detail in Chapters 1 and 2, and propounded them throughout this book.

In contrast to STDP, BIPD assumes that *no* psychodynamic forces are necessary preconditions for depression; such forces are ubiquitous. There is no presumption of an ego defect or personality flaw that is causally related to depression. BIPD understands that dynamic conflicts may lead to short-term emotional upheavals or longer-term personality adaptations or maladaptations. Furthermore, dynamic forces are likely to shape the manifestations of depression when it appears. Regression is seen as an inevitable product of depression, not its cause. Depression causes personality disturbance, but personality disturbance leads to "upset" and *not* depressive illness. Life stressors can contribute to the development of depression or can be consequences of depression.

Although BIPD acknowledges that long-standing negative cognitive perceptions can lead to depressive mood, it makes an important distinction between a depressive mood that is transient and reversible, and an autonomous depressed mood that is a manifestation of a depressive illness. BIPD sees mood as driving cognition rather than vice versa. BIPD views an individual's cognitive set as existing on a continuum and as extremely mood-responsive, in contrast to CBT, which sees cognition as a more constant though influenceable variable. BIPD recognizes that early life experiences (including depression) can result in negatively oriented thinking, and that this inclination will compound a person's problems when a depressive illness is superimposed on it.

Finally, BIPD makes no assumptions regarding primary interpersonal maladaptation as a cause for depression. Certainly relationship disturbances or disruptions can precipitate depression in vulnerable individuals. Furthermore, we have written extensively about the relationship of grief to depression—namely, that grief and depression are not continuous processes; that grief commonly precipitates depression; and that depression often recruits and intensifies residual grief experiences (Shuchter, 1986; Shuchter & Zisook, 1986, 1990; Zisook & Shuchter, 1993). Both IPT and BIPD appreciate the numerous relationship problems that are direct consequences of depression.

GOALS AND IMPLEMENTATION OF PSYCHOTHERAPY

In psychodynamic psychotherapy, the relief of depression is viewed as a secondary consequence of a more primary goal: understanding previously unconscious conflict, especially conflict pertaining to the losses that have "caused" the depression (Freud, 1915/1957). A patient should develop insight into the mechanisms of defense that have hidden these conflicts from view; relive the emotional experiences of loss, disappointment, and rage; work through unrealistic narcissistic strivings for unabated love or admiration; and obtain some symptomatic relief through modification of primitive and demanding superego structures (Strupp & Binder, 1984; Luborsky, 1984; Jacobson, 1971). Different forms of STDP, as well as longer-term dynamic therapies, emphasize different aspects of these goals.

Mann (1973) uses a model of time-limited psychotherapy (12 sessions) that emphasizes the patients' struggle with the treatment's paradigm. According to Mann, when patients are confronted with the reality that all of their hopes and needs cannot be met by the therapist, and with their fears that they cannot face the adult world alone, they will experience and work through the narcissistic injury, loss, and rage that their lost childhoods represent. Davanloo's (1978) approach utilizes a flexible but abbreviated exploratory mode that is highly confrontational of patients' defensive operations, and that moves quickly toward interpretations linking transference resistances with the patients' past relationships and current relationships. Sifneos's (1979) anxiety-provoking form of STDP is another highly active and interpretive approach; it examines traditional Oedipal conflicts as the course of symptomatic distress. All of these approaches assume the same etiology and utilize the same methods to achieve their goals of insight and personality modification, regardless of the symptomatic disorder they may be treating. It is believed that symptoms will resolve once the underlying conflicts are solved; in this sense, STDP purports to be curative.

CBT (e.g., Beck et al., 1979) aims to provide symptomatic relief from depression through a systematic effort to change depressed individuals' automatic and maladaptive ways of thinking and behaving. Patients learn to direct their thoughts and behaviors in more positive ways—first by identifying those patterns that are maladaptive; then by learning the erroneous assumptions that underlie such patterns; and finally by practicing and applying thoughts and behaviors that are more positive and adaptive in regard to themselves, their lives and relationships, and their futures. To the extent that this restructuring is successful, CBT should also be curative.

IPT (Klerman et al., 1984) pursues both symptomatic relief and improvements in relationships and social skills. IPT tries to achieve this by having patients examine problems within their existing family relationships, work through their losses, improve communication with their spouses/partners or family members, and pursue individual social skills training as needed. To the extent that IPT is seen by its proponents as palliative and adjunctive, rather than curative, it can be combined with pharmacotherapy in a way that is theoretically consistent with its conception of psychopathology.

The goals of BIPD are (1) to provide an educational and supportive structure within which medical treatment of depression can proceed with the greatest efficiency; and (2) through educating patients and helping them to understand the effects of depression on all aspects of their lives, to maximize their effectiveness in and satisfaction with living. Included in both of these goals are assumptions about the importance of significant others as informants, monitors, and sources of support. As a means of improving the quality of that support, a patient's significant others are also educated about the language of depression as it is expressed in their relationship with the patient, in order to minimize the effects of distortions. An important objective of all exploration and education in BIPD is to achieve an understanding of how the language of depression leads to potentially maladaptive and/or destructive moral imperatives, which should be actively opposed by therapist, patient, and significant others.

In contrast with psychodynamic treatments, BIPD offers no cure. Personality change is achieved in BIPD by controlling depression with medication and reversing those state-dependent regressive personality characteristics that have emerged with depression. There are no primary assumptions about maladaptive personality structure in BIPD; what patients are to achieve insight into is the continuum of mood-related personality states. "Insight" is not defined by achieving understanding only in the absence of symptoms: Patients with depression can have both healthy personality structures and deep personal insight and can still be "sick" with depression, much as they might be with cancer. Insight into psychodynamic forces in BIPD is yet another means of education about the language of depression, as patients recognize the regression produced by mood changes and the forms such regression can take.

The goals of BIPD resemble some of the goals of CBT, particularly its efforts to correct distorted thinking and behavior. However, in BIPD such distortions are understood as products of depression's impact on the continuum of thoughts and behaviors in the patient's repertoire. There is not a wholesale dismissal of the validity of negative thinking and behavior, but rather an examination of the developmental origins of both negative and positive cognitions and behaviors as they appear in different mood states. For example, self-criticism has "legitimate" roots in parental criticism and personal experiences of failure or inadequacy, and has its appropriate place in a continuum moving toward self-confidence or even self-aggrandizement. In BIPD, these anchor points are understood as living homeostatically in some balance that is highly mood-dependent. Depression yields a hypertrophy of self-criticism. In BIPD this is seen as a distortion, and efforts by both therapist and patient are directed toward reestablishing homeostasis. In CBT, by contrast, the patient may be encouraged to strive for, rehearse, and accept a predominant and "justified" view of self-confidence. Both BIPD and CBT encourage a presentation of and behavior consistent with self-confidence. Similarly, both BIPD and CBT encourage behavioral efforts directed at activity, productive engagement, and positive thinking.

Although involvement of significant others and attention to interpersonal behavior are important in BIPD, BIPD differs from IPT in viewing interpersonal pathology predominantly as a consequence and not as a cause of depression. In BIPD, there is no presumption that depressed patients have *primary* interpersonal dysfunctions or inhibitions. If such a dysfunction exists, it will be identified, and psychotherapeutic efforts may address such problems. However, treating these problems or other targets of IPT (e.g., losses, transitional states, or life stressors) is "incidental" or "ancillary" in BIPD; successful negotiation of such issues will enhance patients' quality of life, but will not necessarily have any impact on their illness. BIPD is more concerned with helping patients to understand how such circumstances will complicate their depression, make the manifestations of depressive phenomena more camouflaged, or press the patients toward maladaptive moral imperatives.

PSYCHOTHERAPEUTIC TECHNIQUES AND PRACTICES

In psychodynamic psychotherapies, techniques and practices have evolved in many ways; they range from open-ended and highly regressive approaches at one end of the continuum to more highly structured, time-limited, and focused approaches at the other. Central to the practical techniques of STDP and longer-term psychodynamic psychotherapies are the uses of expressive, cathartic, and empathic modes of interaction between patient and therapist; examination and confrontation of a patient's defenses and resistances, including transference resistance; repeated observation, clarification, and "working through" of the patient's distortions; and the fullest uncovering of the patient's unconscious (Greenson, 1967).

In CBT, therapy is a standardized and systematic series of learning experiences, with regular review of previous sessions and intervening cognitions and behaviors (Beck et al., 1979). Patients are taught to recognize and record "depressogenic" cognitions and behaviors. The beliefs underlying these are systematically explored and challenged; alternative beliefs are then offered and practiced as homework. Over time, through effort and repetition, these more adaptive views will be incorporated into the processes of automatic thinking and behavior. Assertiveness training and role rehearsal provide additional means of enhancing social skills and positive self-cognitions. All of these processes encourage activity to counteract depression's passivity.

IPT emphasizes the solving of interpersonal problems (Klerman et al., 1984). Educational techniques are utilized initially to deal with overt depressive symptoms. There is a full examination both of the symptomatic picture and of the life events and interpersonal problems that are deemed to contribute to the disorder. Patients are given information, including literature, about depression as a clinical condition. A treatment plan will focus on one of the central paradigms of IPT: loss, interpersonal role disputes, role transitions, or interpersonal deficits. The most relevant theme or themes are then explored in the here and now. Efforts are made to help patients improve their communication skills, achieve perspective in important relationships, improve their social skills, and examine losses and accompanying affects.

The techniques and practices of BIPD incorporate elements of all of the major psychotherapeutic approaches. These include education; symptom review and monitoring; examination of the language of depression; challenges to the moral imperatives that are generated by the illness; empathic understanding of the many forms of suffering in depression; and coping skills exploration and training.

Like STDP and other forms of psychodynamic psychotherapy, BIPD incorporates developmental exploration and interpretation. Interpretations in BIPD, however, are of a very different nature than in STDP. They are focused on helping a patient (1) understand developmental dynamics as a means of appreciating the current language of regression and its distortive potential; (2) learn about the long-term developmental effects of lifelong depression; (3) understand what developmental trauma may have enhanced or sensitized a preexisting predisposition to depression; or (4) empathically explore the illness of a parent, which may have contributed to the patient's experience of deprivation, neglect, or abuse in childhood. This exploration is *not* directed at determining the etiology of depression for the purposes of working through the unresolved and unconscious conflicts that are deemed to have caused it and sustained it, as in STDP.

Like CBT, BIPD seeks to correct cognitive distortions both to improve a patient's mood whenever possible, and, more importantly, to prevent the other consequences of distorted cognitions and behaviors as these get played out interpersonally, functionally, and intrapsychically. Both CBT and BIPD encourage and support structured activity as an antidote to depression's paralysis.

Unlike IPT, BIPD does not assume the existence of interpersonal problems that are unrelated to the consequences of depression. When a patient has interpersonal problems, exploration of these, the enhancement of communication skills, and resolution of conflict are incorporated into the treatment. Most interpersonal work in BIPD, however, is focused on clarifying and minimizing the role of depression in causing such conflict.

THE PATIENT–THERAPIST RELATIONSHIP

In STDP and other psychodynamic therapies (Strupp et al., 1982; Karasu, 1977), the patient–therapist relationship is central to the processes of change that are sought. The psychotherapeutic alliance reflects the ongoing collaboration between patient and therapist in achieving the goals of treatment—in this instance, personality change through understanding; insight into defenses; and adaptive maturation. Through the elaboration and intensification of transference, and in psychoanalysis through the development and examination of the transference neurosis, patients reexperience elements of earlier critical relationships; this gives them opportunities to study their responses, and to reconsider and rework older patterns of relating. In order to facilitate the emergence of patients' projections and other transference phenomena, the therapist presents himself or herself in neutral fashion. However, as in all thera-pies, the therapist's availability, reliability, empathy, and concern pro-vide the matrix of emotional support that allows other aspects of treat-ment to proceed. In addition, the patient incorporates these elements over time, first as positive external mirrors and eventually as parts of his or her self-concept. Identification with the therapist is a concept cen-tral to change and defines yet another aspect of the patient–therapist relationship.

The relationship between patient and therapist in CBT relies upon the establishment and maintenance of a positive transference, in which the power and expertise of the therapist are utilized to direct the patient's work. There is a very active collaboration, with continual feedback from therapist to patient. The two process each depressive thought or behav-ior as a phenomenon to be studied, as a hypothesis to be tested and challenged, and as a stimulus for a new form of cognition. The therapist plays an active teaching role with the patient (Beck et al., 1979; Rush, 1982).

In IPT (Klerman et al., 1984), the therapist is not a neutral figure, but an active advocate for the patient. The therapist's functions are variably exploratory and directive, operating on the level of a positive transference. Although there is no intentional use of the transference as a subject of exploration and study, as in psychodynamic psychotherapy, the patient's responses to the therapist may be utilized in IPT in dealing with issues of grief or interpersonal disputes, or the therapist may be used as a model by a patient with social skills deficits.

As described in Chapter 6, the patient–therapist relationship in BIPD is based upon a continuing positive alliance and advocacy. As in psychodynamic therapy, the therapist is empathic and encourages ex-pression and exploration, albeit toward a different end—that is, toward elaboration of the manifestations of depression, as compared to the de-velopment of greater regression and insight for its own sake in psycho-dynamic therapy. Examination of transference material may occur in BIPD as a means of appreciating issues of dependency, inadequacy, and frustration with ineffective treatment. Again, however, BIPD eschews the heuristic value of such insight in favor of its application to under-standing and coping with the effects of depression.

As in CBT, the patient–therapist relationship in BIPD relies heavily on the expertise of the therapist in an educational and collaborative al-liance. The emphases of the education are somewhat different, but both depend upon fostering a positive and limited degree of dependency.

The roles of the therapist in IPT and BIPD are closely parallel, par-ticularly insofar as both forms of psychotherapy have been designed to be integrated with psychopharmacological treatment. Both treatments demand flexibility in the therapist as explorer and director—roles that are often complicated further in cases where a physician may be prescribing and treating psychotherapeutically.

LIMITATIONS AND POTENTIALLY HARMFUL EFFECTS

From a biological perspective, all forms of psychotherapy for depression that have evolved from nonbiological concepts of psychopathology are inherently flawed. The flaws begin as conceptual ones, but translate quickly into practical ones. Such conceptual and practical errors may have trivial or serious consequences.

STDP and other forms of psychodynamic psychotherapy have several potential detrimental consequences:

1. Psychodynamic therapy treats symptoms instead of the underlying disorder. To the extent that the language of depression translates into interpersonal, functional, and self-conceptual issues, the clinician who treats such personality-related issues as the primary problems is addressing the artifacts of depression rather than the actual disorder. This is an ironic 180-degree reversal of the longer-standing notion that medical treatment of depression is treatment of the symptoms rather than the underlying disorder.

2. As a corollary, these misconceptions about what is wrong with the patient will lead to errors in diagnosis and to incorrect treatment. It has been standard practice among dynamic psychotherapists to see primary depressive disorders as symptomatic of deeper problems. Since all people are normally conflicted about most areas of living, and these conflicts are heightened in the regression that accompanies depression, there are unlimited opportunities to assess depression as a personality disorder and thus to fail to treat it. At least half of the thousands of depressed patients we have seen over the years have been misdiagnosed and mistreated because of such errors.

3. Time is used quite inefficiently in dynamic therapies for depression. Inordinate amounts of time are spent dealing with issues that are minimally relevant to either the etiology or treatment of depression. Mechanisms that are assumed to be "causal" on the basis of unsubstantiated theory become the foci for exhaustive psychological work. For example, an adult with lifelong depression may come to believe that parental neglect is responsible for the depression, or the therapist will interpret retroflexed anger at parental neglect as the cause. Endless hours may then be spent examining this issue as it "recurs" in every facet of

daily living, in each reaction to the therapist, and in every experience of frustration. There may be little consideration of whether the patient's anger is a *product* of depression; of whether the perception of neglect itself is a reflection of childhood depression manifested as a heightened sense of criticism, an intensified neediness, or a distortion of others' motives; or of the likelihood that despite whatever may have contributed to depression, it now has a "life of its own" that is dissociated from its causes, so that even if the patient had the power to undo earlier events (which of course is not the case), the depression would remain.

4. Psychodynamic psychotherapy posits that the ultimate control of the illness is in the hands of the patient. The depression is a product of the patient's unresolved conflicts and inadequate personality strength (defenses). "Where id was, there let ego be" suggests that patients have the capacity, through insight and perseverance, to cure their depression. This is not true. Furthermore, patients whose symptomatology persists in the face of "adequate" psychotherapy are considered self-defeating, are viewed as resistant to treatment, and are ultimately blamed for their continued suffering. It is a rare patient who doesn't start out feeling responsible for his or her illness; assumptions such as those of psychodynamic theory confirm such feelings.

5. Because the natural history of depression is one of recurrence, patients who are treated with psychotherapy and feel "cured" by the psychological work they have done are almost inevitably disappointed and self-deprecating when they experience another depressive episode. They assume that they have done insufficient work in their earlier treatment or that their previously identified and improving conflicts have grown worse again, causing the return of the depression. There is no recognition that depression is likely to recur regardless of what psychological intervention occurs. There is also little realization that a depressive episode may resolve without any intervention. Such a resolution is likely to be deemed illusory when no psychological work addressing "underlying conflicts" has been done.

6. Psychotherapy that is regressively oriented is probably contraindicated in depressed patients. The regression of depression needs no help in worsening (see discussion in Chapter 6).

7. Dynamic therapies' emphasis on nondirectiveness and the promotion of self-understanding assumes that the findings of patients' self-explorations are valid and real. Accurate empathy reinforces the perceptive distortions of depressed persons. The dynamic therapist's encouragement of self-understanding further validates such distortions and may lead patients to act on the basis of these views. For example, depressed persons may "discover" while regressed that their work is not a "calling" or that their choice of a spouse or partent was based on the "wrong" motives. Without a concept of state-dependent distortion, the biologi-

cally uninformed therapist will have no grounds for advising such patients that their decisions may be incorrect. Although a dynamic therapy
may be nondirective, its initial conditions may dictate that patients make
no major changes during therapy. This condition may have little power
in the face of depressive imperatives, and a therapist committed to nondirectiveness may not be able to intervene, other than to interpret such
acting out as resistance to treatment—an interpretation that will increase
the patients' self-reproach.

8. Psychodynamic psychotherapy may undermine the support systems of depressed individuals. When the above-mentioned distortions
lead depressed patients to end relationships, the passive acceptance of
these "insights" or similar insights about important relationships, institutional attachments, and other affiliations may result in the patients'
being deprived of their supports at a time when they need them most.

CBT for depression has as its major drawback the belief that depressive illness is invariably the consequence of faulty cognitions and
behaviors. Although there are patients whose milder depressive states
respond well to this approach, total adherence to the belief places an
enormous, unfulfillable responsibility upon those patients with moderate to severe depression who do not respond to the approach. They believe that their thinking and behavior cause the depression, and that their
thinking and behavior should cure it.

Empirical research (Rush et al., 1977) has demonstrated that the
combination of CBT and pharmacotherapy has an advantage over either "pure" approach in the treatment of depression. This finding is quite
consistent with the theoretical orientation of BIPD, but not with that of
CBT. Although this inconsistency may not seem very problematic for
practitioners of CBT ("If it works, use it!"), patients are left confused
and still burdened by the ideas that they control their depression and
are "unsuccessful" if they need medication.

IPT for depression, designed as an adjunctive treatment with psychopharmacology (Klerman et al., 1984), has many areas of overlap with
BIPD: recognition of depression as a medical disorder, and patient education based on this recognition; incorporation of significant others in
treatment; and attention to the consequences of depression for relationships. At the same time, however, IPT emphasizes four interpersonal
paradigms as *causal* in the development of depression, and proposes substantial psychotherapeutic work to address and minimize these "causes":
grief, interpersonal disputes, role transitions, and interpersonal deficits.
As extensions of elements of traditional psychoanalytic beliefs, these "associational" connections to depression are elevated to explanations of
psychopathology and are incorporated into patients' derogatory views of
themselves. It leaves the door wide open for patients (and their fami-

lies) to assume the blame for their illness. Troubled relationships may make life hard, and certainly make the impact of depression worse, but problems in relationships are more likely to be secondary to the depression than to cause it.

Our argument is not with the focus upon interpersonal stressors or limitations, which may or may not be relevant and useful areas in which to help the afflicted and their families understand and cope with depression. It is with the assumptions that these factors are etiologically central, and that working through or eradicating them will protect patients from future depression. Interpersonal competence may mitigate against the pitfalls associated with depression; stronger relationships will provide support against depression's attacks; grief intensifies in the face of depression. However, interpersonal "perfection" will not prevent depression in a vulnerable individual whose time has come.

People who have suffered from depression are hungry for knowledge about what will protect them from recurrence. All psychologically based theories of the etiology of depression create this illusion: "If you fix this psychological flaw, you will be protected." There is no scientific basis for such a belief, though one therapy with a partial psychological explanation, IPT, has demonstrated an effect upon delaying (not preventing) recurrence of depression (Kupfer et al., 1992).

BIPD brings its own problems to patients struggling with depression. First, by undermining the notion that patients will be able to control their destinies through correct, professionally guided techniques and through their own will and effort, BIPD will cause some patients to feel even more demoralized and out of control than they were before. The idea that depression is a biological illness is likely to be experienced as a narcissistic injury—the identification of another kind of flaw, albeit a flaw of nature. Second, patients who have made major investments in other forms of treatment often feel disillusioned, angered, and betrayed by both their former and their present therapists, especially when biologically uninformed therapists may not have referred them for or may have actively discouraged them from receiving medical treatments that subsequently prove to be effective. Such feelings may diminish the value of otherwise useful treatment by otherwise caring and well-intended therapists.

Although both of these potentially detrimental consequences are common, patients will adapt to the first as they see their own progress and to the second as they came to appreciate the natural course of all scientific progress. The acquisition of the latest version of "the truth" is not always easy. However, the same is true of depression as it is of heart disease: Revealing the diagnosis to a patient may be traumatic or upsetting, but such a step is essential if the person is to understand the illness and get the proper treatment.

·8·

Case Examples

In this chapter, we present a number of detailed case examples of the use of BIPD. Each of these examples represents a variation or series of variations on the central themes of treatment. Our purpose is to demonstrate the clinical thinking that determines both general strategies and specific applications based on the unique characteristics presented by patients. We proceed from the more straightforward and simple types of cases to the more complex and demanding ones. All of these patients were diagnosed as having major depressive disorder and/or dysthymic disorder.

CASE 1: MARY

Mary was a single woman in her 40s, a career administrator at a university, when she presented for treatment of her depression. She had been treated fairly continually for recurrent major depression for the previous 10 years; much of this treatment had been managed by her internist. She said that when she was taking an antidepressant, she was fine: She enjoyed her work, performed well, had numerous friends, and treasured her solitude to pursue other interests. When she was off antidepressants, she experienced depressed mood, lowered energy, sleep disturbances, anhedonia, and compromised work functioning. Over the years, she had been tried on numerous antidepressants, and trazodone had been found to be most effective. The only side effect of any significance caused by the trazodone was some mild cognitive slowing (she wasn't as "quick" as usual in her thinking).

Mary's developmental history was without significant trauma. She had grown up in an intact middle-class family that had some depression on her mother's side. Mary was always quiet but sociable, with a small cadre of friends. A good student, she completed college and graduate school, and soon afterward began working at the university.

Mary demonstrated confidence about herself, satisfaction with her work, and pleasure in her relationships. She believed that her depressive proclivities were genetic in origin and biological in nature, and that they did not represent anything "wrong" with her. She had adopted the view that her taking an antidepressant was like a diabetic's taking insulin, and she was quite matter-of-fact about her need for continued pharmacological treatment.

The psychiatrist who treated her agreed with Mary's own assessment that she was a healthy, adaptive woman who would need continued antidepressant treatment indefinitely. After 10 years with repeated efforts to discontinue the treatment, it seemed unlikely that the underlying depression would remit spontaneously. There was no indication of a need for psychotherapy, since the patient was well educated about depression in general and *her* depression in particular; she had no significant developmental problems as a result of living with her depression; her functioning and coping skills were excellent; she never lost perspective or was "captured" by her depression; and most of the time her depression was fully controlled with antidepressants.

Treatment consisted of increasingly prolonged intervals between sessions; the sessions went from monthly to quarterly to annual checkups, with the understanding that any perturbations within Mary's life could be dealt with on an as-needed basis. Because of the problematic side effect of cognitive slowing that Mary experienced with trazodone, she and the psychiatrist had periodic discussions about whether to initiate treatment with another antidepressant to lessen or eliminate this effect. After 4 years, a trial of fluoxetine yielded continued full control of her depression and the return of her cognitive "sharpness." At this writing, she remains on a regimen of fluoxetine and of yearly sessions with this supportive message: "Antidepressants control your depression—you know how to live your life."

Mary represents a large number of people whose chronic depression is controllable with an antidepressant, who have come to recognize and accept their illness, and who seem to understand its effects and pursue intervention. They require little psychotherapy and infrequent monitoring. Therapists should always be aware that such situations can change: People may become refractory or intolerant to some drugs; medical problems can exacerbate depression or change people's tolerance of antidepressants; the depression may take a more virulent course; patients who have never been "captive" may become so. As a result, some form of monitoring should always take place.

CASE 2: JIM

Jim, an executive of a major corporation, first came for treatment at age 49. He developed major depression in the context of a corporate takeover, which involved the disruption and upheaval of policies that he had developed and that had made the company successful. He was stripped of some of his authority and reassigned to work he had done years before. He was understandably humiliated and furious, and gradually over several months became more depressed. He developed insomnia with frequent awakenings; an increase in his appetite, with a 40-pound weight gain and continual nervous eating; anergy, against which he struggled to maintain his work output because of a fear of failure; complete anhedonia and loss of libido; distractibility and impaired concentration; and unending ruminations. The most distressing symptom for Jim was a sharp increase in irritability: He became easily annoyed and had critical outbursts toward his two sons. This loss of control at home in particular, the general feeling of being out of control, were what brought him to treatment. He was never suicidal.

Jim was the older of two siblings in a solid, close-knit, well-to-do family. He had generally been a happy child, very popular and a good student. He became a star athlete in high school and college, and had a short-lived career as a professional athlete before joining the corporation, in which he rose quickly to positions of greater responsibility and authority until he became one of its chief exercutive officers (CEOs). Until the recent takeover, Jim had loved his work and devoted much time and energy to it.

Jim had met his wife in college; they had been married 27 years and had two sons in college. Jim and his wife (who accompanied him to his first session) agreed that they'd had an excellent marriage and Jim had been a good father, finding time for his sons' development and being quite active in their sports activities. It was clear to both spouses that he was "not himself."

Jim had had no prior psychiatric contact. There was no history of depression, alcoholism or other mental disorder in his family. His health had generally been good, except for occasional cluster headaches treated intermittently with propranolol (a beta-adrenergic blocking agent that can produce some depression with continued use). He rarely used alcohol and never used other drugs.

Upon further assessment, it became clear that Jim had little understanding about depression. A sophisticated and bright man in most respects, he realized that much of his turmoil, frustration, humiliation, anger, and diminished sense of control were precipitated by the seizure of power in his corporation by "outsiders." What he couldn't fathom was the discrepancy between his usual high level of functioning and the present impairment to his thinking, feelings, and behavior. This loss of control over himself was anathema and shameful to him. His private humiliation was bearable, but his outbursts toward his sons left him with shame that pushed him to seek help. He felt weak, dependent, and in-adequate—"like a wimp," as he put it.

Jim accepted the clinician's explanations about depression, though he was more appreciative of the reassurance that his depression could be helped. A medical assessment revealed no abnormalities, and he was started on amitriptyline, which helped his sleep immediately. After 2 weeks of antidepressant treatment, Jim was feeling somewhat better and was no longer as irritable and "on edge" with his family. Over the following month his depression largely lifted, leaving some residual dimin-ished libido and a mild dry mouth (an amitriptyline side effect).

In considering psychotherapy for Jim, the clinician weighed the following factors. On the one hand, it was clear that he needed educa-tion about depression and its effects on his relationships, work, and sense of self, primarily as a means of monitoring his state of depression. On the other hand, none of these areas presented any significant risk within Jim's life because of his personal strengths, adaptive skills, and wealth of good will from others. His personal qualities of ambition, self-control, hard work, and determination were effective enough to override most of the functionally reactive elements of his depression. He was able to hold much of his irritability in check even at home, and certainly always did so at work. His application of more time and more effort, a baseline of high intelligence, and familiarity with and skills in conducting his job resulted in minimal loss of efficiency, despite his impaired concentration, distractibility, diminished interest, loss of motivation, and anergy. Edu-cation would help him achieve perspective about the process and lessen the impact of depression on his self-esteem, which had already come under attack with the corporate restructuring.

Over the course of six sessions of psychotherapy and 3 months, Jim was, with the exception of some continued diminished libido, "back to his old self." He was uncritically accepting of his treatment, especially as it had been so effective. Although he understood the impact and language of his own depression, he was more interested in the "bottom line" of treatment—results (i.e., how he felt). He and the therapist dis-cussed the idea of his staying on the antidepressant for a full 6 months, and he was agreeable. Furthermore, he was "vindicated" at work: His re-placement did poorly and was fired, and Jim was invited to return as a CEO. This helped him beyond the already established remission of his symptoms.

Jim returned for treatment 1 year after he left. Six months after discontinuing his antidepressant, he began to have a recurrence of symp-toms of the same nature, but worse than before. He became increasingly preoccupied with work-related issues, and, for the first time ever, began ruminating about *not* committing suicide. Because of the time frame and absence of any specific stressors, this episode was considered as an exacerbation and continuation of his index episode of major depression.

It was disconcerting to learn that Jim had again gone for several months in a state of progressive depression without seeking help, especially as he had responded so well to amitriptyline the first time. When the therapist explored this with Jim, it became clear that although Jim did realize that the depression had reappeared (i.e., despite its powerful impact, he was not a "captive" of the depression), he maintained the stance that he would fight against it on his own. He felt that his manhood was at stake, and he fought against the depression until it was sufficiently out of control that he couldn't tolerate it any longer.

Once again, Jim was placed on amitriptyline; he was substantially better at 1 month and in full remission by 2 months. A second set of six psychotherapy sessions focused largely on the issue of his being able to accept that he had a vulnerability to depression that he could not control. This reality is terribly difficult for many patients to accept, and Jim's willingness to entertain this notion ran contrary to his powerful pride and need for control. He became more able to consider this because of the potential benefit: Early intervention for the exacerbation could have saved him 3 or 4 months of suffering. Treatment proceeded to focus on his acceptance of this vulnerability.

In treatment, such a patient's pride and need for control as impediments to an acceptance of vulnerability can be explored, on the one hand, from an individual, idiosyncratic developmental perspective, in which the threads of these themes can be traced to their manifestations at various milestones. On the other hand, they can be understood quite efficiently and effectively as universal dynamic themes that have predominantly adaptive functions, and yet maladaptive potential. Confirming the strength of such characteristics, and empathizing with the problems they may create, may be useful means of educating patients who are "resistant." As Jim's therapist told him, "Jim, your pride and need to stay in control have pushed you and helped you to accomplish a lot. Right now they seem to stand in the way of your being able to appreciate the power of your depression."

The therapist's acknowledgment of the adaptive elements contained in all dynamic conflicts helps patients accept the maladaptive features that are part of the "package." It can lessen the defensiveness that is often an automatic reaction to the identification of "pathological" features, as patients so often interpret therapists' observations. The matter-of-fact identification of these normal aspects of human nature further mitigates against such patients' perception of their unhealthiness. It is especially important to emphasize "normalizing" rather than "pathologizing" elements in people who must contend with the reality that they have a biological "defect."

CASE 3: LINDA

Linda, an accomplished scientist in her 40s who had been married over 20 years and was the mother of two, came for treatment in the midst of a major depressive episode of several months' duration. At the time of her presentation, she was feeling overwhelmed and tortured by the severity of her state of mind, and was frightened by fleeting passive fantasies of being dead. She had marked sleep and appetite disturbances, anergy, anhedonia, a loss of resilience, irritability, impaired cognition, and marked self-deprecation. She ruminated incessantly about how she was a failure as a wife and mother, a pretender as a scientist, and a generally worthless person. An extraordinarily hard-working and perfectionist woman by nature, Linda persisted in all of her roles, exerting even greater than usual effort in the face of her depression; however, she was unable to experience any satisfaction anywhere, beyond her awareness that she was able to "keep her head above water." Her driven nature precluded any consideration of acting upon the distorting and disruptive influences of depression on her work, relationships, or self.

Linda had first experienced an episode of major depression in college. There had been two or three other episodes, occurring with increasing frequency, in her 30s (postpartum); in recent years, a dysthymic state (or incompletely resolved major depression—they may be the same) had evolved. Her "lifeline" of depression is shown in Figure 6.1 (see p. 132).

Linda was in good health. She did not drink or use drugs. Her family history was positive for depression in her brother, who had been successfully treated with antidepressants. Linda had been in psychotherapy and couple therapy within 2 years of her presentation; both of these therapies were supportive and helpful to her in coping with the day-to-day problems created by depression. However, in her mind, the psychotherapies tended to reinforce the notions that she was "really screwed up" and personally responsible for her plight because of her personality and the way she viewed things.

Linda had read extensively about depression, particularly in the psychological literature. She had applied herself to learning cognitive therapy, but as hard as she tried (and she was a woman with remarkable work habits), she benefited very little from this approach. She was able to undermine any positive thought with a critical one; as a result, she felt still worse about herself. She was inclined to take any information and use it to reinforce her self-deprecation.

Linda was the first-born of two siblings in a middle-class family. Her mother was a very demanding, cruel, self-centered woman who dominated a caring, passive husband and their children. Linda experienced her mother as a woman who was unrelentingly harsh and critical, competitive rather than nurturing; yet the mother had a vision of herself as giving all to her family. Her cruelty was largely emotional in nature. As hard as Linda tried to please her mother throughout her life, she was met with direct taunts or with implications that she was bad, stupid, and ugly. Linda's strivings for perfection yielded great accomplishments; however, her mother experienced most of these not as things to be proud of, but as seemingly demeaning affronts to her, and she retaliated with abuse. The mother viewed Linda's accomplishments positively only if they could enhance her own image before others, and even then any outward expression of pride was reserved for the suitable audience. Linda found some immediate comfort with both her brother and father, but she was disappointed by her father's inability to protect her from her mother.

During adolescence, Linda met her future husband. They were "soulmates" who sought a haven in each other and who grew up together. Allan's eyes reflected the goodness, beauty, and brilliance that Linda had sought from her mother; within the safety and affection of their relationship, both spouses thrived in their marriage, family, and careers. Linda had already developed her intellectual life as a sanctuary from bad feelings, as a source of accomplishment to bolster her vulnerable self-esteem, and (most importantly) as an independently satisfying pursuit over which she had full ownership.

The developmental picture just described emerged over time in psychotherapy. At the time of Linda's presentation, her depression was sufficiently severe that the first order of business was to alleviate her symptoms. This was essential both for inherent humanitarian reasons and for purposes of further assessment under circumstances that were not so strongly influenced by the state of her depression. "Let's try and understand who you are when you're not depressed" is one way of conveying this to such a patient.

Linda was treated with nortriptyline, which quickly helped her sleep and anxiety. Two weeks later, her mood, energy, capacity for pleasure, work efficiency, and outlook were improving substantially. The depression was in almost full remission after 5 weeks of treatment. She experienced an enormous sense of relief that she was not doomed to live her life in the tortured state to which she had become accustomed. Despite her vast knowledge of science, she had never allowed herself to consider depression a medical disorder, because it would have been an "easy way out." She had remained convinced that the "root" of her depression lay in her developmental problems and personality, and that these could not be altered. She remained unconvinced that this wasn't true, but her response to treatment was undeniable.

As her depression cleared, the following formulation emerged as a guide for psychotherapy. Linda always carried with her the vulnerability to her self-esteem that had been forged by her mother's narcissism and cruelty. This vulnerability was held in check by the views of her husband, feedback from her work, and occasional self-endorsements—all of which could be subverted by stressful circumstances on a short-term basis, and annihilated by almost any degree of depression. This all-encompassing self-deprecation contributed substantially to Linda's being "captured" by the depression. She could maintain no continuing perspective that she was in a state of depression, because she saw all of the manifestations of depression as simply reflections of the "reality" that she was worthless as a mother, wife, daughter, and scientist, and in fact deserving of the suffering she experienced. Whan Linda was assessed for risks, it was clear that she had enormous internal resources that allowed her to function at all times, and superego demands that would not permit her to "give in." As severe as her depression had ever been, there had never been a realistic concern that it could cost Linda her career, family, or life. The only risk generated by the depression was that of continued personal suffering.

The primary goal of psychotherapy, therefore, became largely to have Linda achieve an enduring insight into the interactions between her developmentally determined vulnerability and the state-dependent features of this vulnerability—interactions that would put her at risk for suffering depression and not seeking out an intervention that had already been established as effective. Another related goal was to help her improve her nondepressed self-esteem, which was better than her self-esteem during depression, but still impaired. Because of the excellent control of her depression achieved by antidepressants, and the patient's superior abilities and coping skills, the therapist was soon inclined to begin cutting down the frequency of appointments from weekly to biweekly and probably monthly. However, Linda requested that they continue to meet weekly, to maximize the benefits of psychotherapy. The therapist accepted part of Linda's request at face value, believing that it also reflected some insecurity about her recent gains. He had wished to express a vote of confidence in her by decreasing the frequency of sessions, but could see the usefulness of more intense work.

In regard to the need for continued medication, the therapist said on a number of occasions that it was impossible to know about this at the time of Linda's beginning treatment, but that because of what appeared to be the development of chronicity in recent years, there was a good possibility that antidepressant treatment might be necessary indefinitely. Practically, Linda and the therapist developed a plan to treat the depressive episode continuously until the depression was in full remission for 6 months. At this time, with adequate understanding of the depression and its language, sufficient perspective, and close monitoring, the medication would be gradually discontinued. It was agreed that if her depression returned, pharmacological treatment would resume.

One of the difficulties of conducting a form of psychotherapy that helps people understand, prepare for, and cope with depression is that the techniques must be applied at periods of depression in order to be tested fully, and the effectiveness of pharmacological interventions can preclude such opportunities. At times, a treatment plan will include discontinuing medication. This becomes an experiment to see whether a depressive episode is in true remission or whether it has simply been controlled by the drug. The purpose of the experiment is to find out whether the patient is able to go without the medication and still be free of depression. It is not an experiment designed to produce depression so that the patient can "try out" the effectiveness of psychotherapy; that is an insufficient benefit in relationship to the risks of depression.

Nature and circumstances, however, seem to conduct this experiment in many situations: at the onset of an episode; at points of exacerbation of depression; at times when medication is discontinued by design or because of adverse side effects; at points when patients decide on their own to discontinue their medicine; and at times when "breakthrough" depression occurs while the patient is still on a previously effective dose of an antidepressant. Breakthrough depression may be spontaneous or may be driven by acute stressors or internal metabolic processes. It may also reflect a change in the effectiveness of a given dose of an antidepressant because of some inherent and unknown property, or because of a change in the rate of the drug's metabolism in the liver, excretion in the kidneys, binding to other drugs, or distribution to various sites in the brain. Regardless of their nature or origin, these episodes of breakthrough depression will often respond to small changes in the dose of an antidepressant.

In fact, Linda experienced a number of such episodes, each of which responded rapidly (within a few days) to adjustments of medication. These episodes also provided Linda with valuable learning experiences. The first such episode (as is usually the case) was very frightening, challenging the sense of safety and security she experienced while she was protected from her depression. Each episode, however, provided her with a glimpse of the power of depression to undermine her perspective, functional efficiency, and self-concept. While in the midst of such exacerbations she would find herself becoming "captive," saying, "When I feel this way, it seems that this is reality and the antidepressants create the illusion. Maybe this is just the way things are." The therapist, by then with firm experience-based knowledge and a strong alliance, could say, "No, this is depression; this isn't you. You'll be yourself again next week. I guarantee it." This invariably proved to be the case.

Concurrently, work proceeded on Linda's underlying problem with self-esteem. Through exploration, she gained greater insight into her wishes to please her mother, her consistent guilt in the face of her mother's criticism, and her gradual incorporation of this criticism into her self-concept. She feared becoming like her mother, but knew this was not a realistic fear: She loved her children deeply, nurtured them appropriately though not excessively, and was exquisitely sensitive to their needs. Linda came to appreciate and even empathize with what must have been the pain her own mother suffered, but she also recognized that what she herself had been exposed to was undeserved. She felt great compassion both for what she as a little child had suffered and how her mother might be suffering even now, as Linda kept her at arm's length. She was able to test out different ways of expressing herself to her mother, now thousands of miles away; she even became willing to risk exposure of her daughters to her mother, albeit not without the fear that she would be responsible for any bad feelings the girls might experience. She was able to incorporate some of her therapist's positive regard and feelings for her into this evolving view of herself.

Over the course of a year of almost weekly psychotherapy, Linda developed more flexibility around the edges of her perfectionistic strivings. (Of course, as a "good enough" mother and scientist, she still had demands about two standard deviations above the norm.) She recognized that she still had some level of vulnerability, but that she generally felt good about herself and her life. She had come to terms about her relationship with her mother; her marriage was strong; and her work was very productive. When another episode of breakthrough depression occurred somewhat insidiously over a period of 2–3 weeks, she was very disappointed. For the first time, she was explicit in her hope that with substantial resolution of the powerfully disruptive relationship with her mother, in her head and in the world, she would be free of depression and no longer need antidepressants—in other words, that the treatment could make her "more perfect." Although such issues never disappear, Linda has since struggled to make the adjustment to the other reality: "If I need to take an antidepressant to feel this good, I guess I can live with it." She has become able to see herself as a good person with a good (though demanding and stressful) life, and a bad inheritance that can be controlled. This has not kept her from being critical of her vulnerability to depression.

This core of self-criticism and self-demand has been in part responsible for Linda's episodes of breakthrough depression. Linda has always preferred to be on the lowest possible dose of antidepressant medication necessary to control her depression. In this way, she has felt that she has been able to do all that she can do in terms of her personal contribution to managing her illness. These are sentiments that many therapists and patients share. However, Linda has also had some gradual increase in the amount of antidepressant medication necessary for her stability. Because of her reluctance to have a "cushion" or margin of safety in her dosage, she has been more vulnerable to the emergence of breakthrough depression.

Recently, Linda went through a period of almost a year of continuous remission. Her life was happy and productive—too much so, she felt. Without even a glimpse of euphoria or what might be construed as hypomania, Linda lowered her medication. Why? She had gone on a 3-day weekend skiing vacation and had skied all 3 days, thoroughly enjoying herself. She was not plagued at all by not having worked on a single paper or grant, and this "carefree" state upset her. She felt that she had become undisciplined and lazy, and this was an unacceptable state for her. Unfortunately, she then plummeted into a prolonged period of destabilization, including a period of suicidal preoccupation unmitigated by her sense of her children's need for her. Linda began ruminating about ending her life, rationalizing that her children might be "better off" without a mother who was so inadequate. Linda was upset with her therapist for telling her that her suicide would be "the most devastating thing that could happen to your children—something from which they may never recover." She felt even more hopeless after this, since suicide was not an option she could consider. However, the discussion did interrupt the direction of her thinking. When she was no longer a captive of the depression, she expressed appreciation for the therapist's sentiments. As a result of this experience, in which Linda was totally consumed by the state of her mind, she has become more receptive to having some greater margin of safety in the medical management of her depression. She understands that the risks to her life on a minimal dose of medicine are much greater than the risks to her self-image on 10–20% more.

CASE 4: BILL

Bill was a 33-year-old unmarried computer programmer who sought out continuing treatment for his depression, after several years of psychotherapy with an older male psychoanalyst. His reasons for ending his previous treatment, as he described them, were his frustration with the fact that his therapist "never spoke" to him and his perception that he never felt any better.

Bill had been chronically and continuously depressed for several years, and indicated that he had been depressed throughout most of his childhood. The third of four children of a prominent academician father and a gentle homemaking mother, Bill had been a gifted student, but suffered from brooding and a tendency to isolation. As his depression persisted, he became an underachieving "genius" who felt tortured, alienated, and increasingly angry at his parents, particularly his father. He perceived his father as cold, aloof, and controlling; both at that time and later in his life, he blamed his father for how bad he felt, attributing his depression to acts of omission or commission in parenting.

As a teenager, Bill was evaluated by a psychiatrist, diagnosed as having depression, and treated for a while with different TCAs. There seemed to be some benefit of the medications, but the side effects (sedation and constant dry mouth) made him so uncomfortable that he discontinued their use. Hostile transference issues toward the psychiatrist also contributed to the disruption of this treatment. Some years later, he began the unsuccessful course of psychoanalysis mentioned above.

Despite his persistent depression—characterized by depressed and irritable mood, diminished energy and motivation, fatigue and frequent apathy, social withdrawal, and compensatory constriction of affect—Bill was able to persist in school because of his intelligence and curiosity about computers. When he began taking dancing lessons, he learned that strenuous physical exertion could temporarily energize him and improve his mood, and he pursued this interest for many years. Just as he was on the verge of making dance a career, orthopedic problems interfered, forcing him to change his plans and work in the computer field.

To cope with his depression, Bill organized his work to allow him to sleep late. He energized himself with swimming and body surfing. New projects at work and new relationships with women enabled him to override his depression on a temporary basis, but with time he would become bored, lose interest, and wish to change as the depression reasserted itself. Most of the time, however, his depression was of limited severity, so that he remained reactive to novel stimuli.

At the beginning of his current treatment, Bill was working at a defense industry company designing computer programs. His work suffered from the waxing and waning of interest that accompanied his mood. A relationship with a young woman was in a similar state of flux. He saw himself as impaired and unhappy, and as experiencing lassitude, apathy, and fatigue on a daily basis. He was strongly opposed to treatment with antidepressants because of his prior experience of "coercion" and side effects, and clearly wanted psychotherapy to help him cope with his depression. He had no illusions that psychotherapy would be curative.

Over the next year, Bill was seen in weekly psychotherapy that was highly focused on his day-to-day struggle with depression. He came to understand its effects in all areas of his life as he explored his work, his love life, his relationship with his parents, and his self-concept. He correctly perceived the therapist's concern for and regard of him, and became more animated in his sessions.

The patient's increasing insight into the workings of his depression helped to stabilize his life in various ways. The change in his perspective enabled him to see his family in a different light. In particular, he came to view his father as a shy and not very interpersonally competent man struggling to cope with a depressed son. Bill was able to approach him with this view, and they began to grow closer. In addition, Bill developed an awareness of his depression-driven fickleness and became more able to persist within a relationship. He also began to see that it wasn't the nature of his work or his coworkers that made him feel unhappy (though certainly specific situations arose in which this was the case). Finally, in his relationship with his therapist, Bill found comfort and support, as well as a "mirror" that screened out his depression when he looked for himself. From week to week, Bill looked forward to his sessions as a source of understanding and sanctuary, and as a temporary relief from his depression. He remained reactive much of the time, and, like so many people with dysthymic disorder, found himself increasingly dependent upon his treatment to sustain himself.

However, as is almost always the case, his depression persisted. After a year, when Bill was going through a period of more intense depression, his therapist again confronted him (as he had done intermittently throughout the treatment) with the intransigency of the depression on the one hand, and the efficacy of pharmacological treatment on the other. With some insistence, relying on their good therapeutic alliance and Bill's trust in his judgment, the therapist pointed out the numerous avenues that had not been taken pharmacologically, the possible benefits (which could be enormous), and the minimal risks, together with Bill's shared control in making decisions about much of the process. Bill consented, was started on an MAOI, and had an excellent response. He obtained full remission, which has persisted (with minor glitches) over the subsequent 4 years with continued treatment. The effects of his depression on his life largely dissolved. His work and relationships were revitalized; problems arising in either context were inherent to the work or the relationship, rather than colored or driven by an altered mood. What remained were the elements of self-concept that were products of the depression. Whereas Bill had experienced himself as "impaired," he now recognized that he was "vulnerable." This sense of vulnerability, however, was quite acceptable when coupled with the effective control of the illness.

The only substantial residual "problem" was Bill's dependence on the therapist, accompanied by a lack of confidence and self-reliance. This dependency had been an iatrogenic, though crucial, element in Bill's successful treatment. It was necessary and easy for Bill to understand this dynamic in universal (vs. idiosyncratic) terms, and it was dealt with directly by (1) tapering off the frequency of sessions and (2) examining his struggle with both wanting more of the therapist and appreciating his own growing self-reliance and independence.

Over the past 2 years, Bill has obtained a better job and gotten married. He has been symptomatically stable; the therapist has seen him on four occasions, usually in conjunction with his wife to discuss marital difficulties arising from incompatibilities of style.

In Bill, we can see some of the developmental effects of long-standing depression in all areas of functioning. Insight became a necessary tool in educating Bill about the pervasive effects of his depression. The power of the therapeutic relationship enabled him to overcome his resistance to medical treatment. Once the antidepressant medication proved effective, however, very little work was necessary for Bill to "catch up" in his relationships, career, and self-esteem. Once his depression was controlled, he was able to improve his relationships with his family, persevere in developing a committed relationship with a woman, stay involved with his work, and sustain good feelings about himself.

CASE 5: JANET

Janet was a 31-year-old single professional woman when she moved to a new city, in order to continue her relationship with a man whose work had brought him there earlier. She started a job with a new firm and was soon having problems adjusting to both situations. She had been in long-term psychotherapy in the previous city for "self-destructive problems with relationships and separations," as well as depression. She'd had a brief but unsuccessful trial of a TCA. Her complaint at the time she presented for a new course of treatment was that she had "just screwed up her relationship and didn't know why."

What emerged was a picture of chronic low-grade depression, punctuated by acute episodes of more severe symptoms. During dysthymic periods, Janet functioned well at work, using her work as both a distraction and a stimulus. When away from work, she would seek solace in her relationship with her boyfriend, Glen, and other friends, but experienced a general sense of dissatisfaction, malaise, and an inclination toward novelty seeking for stimulation. During periods of major depression, which were accelerating in frequency, she developed marked sleep and appetite disturbances, irritability, anergy, anhedonia, cognitive disruption, intense dependency, self-deprecation, and guilty and suicidal ruminations.

At these latter times, she began to question the meaning of the work she did. She found herself unable to persevere with any but mundane tasks, and wondered whether she should escape to a tropical island where there were no demands. The relative confidence she exuded about her work even when she was mildly depressed disappeared, replaced by intensifying jealousies about others' positions in the power structure and her perceived standing with her superiors. In her most intimate relationship, she regressed markedly, becoming more jealous and possessive, needy, and angry about Glen's unavailability. She felt more vulnerable to his leaving her, more deserving of his doing so, and more hostile because she was so vulnerable. When she was anxious, she would often drink; on more than one such occasion—because she felt desperate and entitled, and her inhibitions were lowered—she had affairs. This became known to her boyfriend. Finally Glen ended the relationship, confirming her worst fears and her conviction that she was self-destructive. This event was what caused her to seek a new course of treatment.

Janet was the older (by several years) of two sisters in a middle-class Midwestern family. As a child, Janet had been close to her mother and the apple of her father's eye. The father died when she was a teenager; the whole family seemed not to recover from this loss, and forged bonds together as survivors. Janet was a good student and had a satisfactory social life, though she developed a stance of counterdependent toughness that intensified later. She met Glen while she was in college and he was a married graduate student with two children. Eventually he divorced his wife; they had planned to marry after Janet followed him to the new city.

During her psychotherapy in the Midwest, Janet had developed much insight into the central dynamic themes of her life. She understood her vulnerability to loss and her compensatory counterdependency. She knew of her reliance on a paternal mirror for certain aspects of her esteem and her resentment of men because of this. She was aware of her Oedipal victory and the consequent guilt. However, her insight into all these issues was useless in the face of her depression. On the contrary, her depression-driven regressions exacerbated the worst, most threatening, most self-deprecating, guiltiest, and most infantile states. Issues that did not intrude into her daily life during periods of emotional stability flooded her when depression intensified.

This was demonstrated once Janet began treatment with antidepressant medication (initially phenelzine, and later fluoxetine). During the initial stages of treatment, much effort went into exploring the relationship between Janet's depression and her work, relationship, and dynamic regressive experiences. Once it seemed clear just how destructive her depression (not she herself) was to her life, pharmacotherapy was instituted.

Janet responded well to phenelzine, though with some side effects, and better to fluoxetine. Weekly sessions changed to a monthly and then to an as-needed basis. She was well informed, accepted her depression, and developed more insight into the complex interactions of her mood, dynamics, and functioning. Several months would go by with minimal contact until an episode of breakthrough depression occurred. Unfortunately for Janet, these episodes would evolve insidiously, leading to some depressive symptoms, some compromised functioning, and usually some "capture." At such times, she would report some existential crisis in her career or in a relationship. The first two times this occurred, the therapist moved in aggressively, telling her that this wasn't "existence" but depression, and that she probably needed a change in the dosage of her medicine. Janet complied, felt better, and over time came to identify the manifestations of mood instability sooner. When breakthroughs recurred, she would come in asking, "Is this life or depression?"

On a few occasions, it turned out to be "life" as Janet ventured more deeply into a new relationship and experienced real conflict-based turmoil. However, in the context of a stable mood, she was quite capable of tolerating the transient turmoil that was inevitable in such a risk. This relationship, worked out essentially on her own, became critical to reestablish a belief that she was not somehow predestined to destroy all relationships—that depression had been a major provocateur in the past. She also adopted a friend and colleague as a monitor—a woman who knew her well enough in both depressed and undepressed states to give her feedback and support.

Janet represents someone whose developmental vulnerabilities and depression converged to create the picture of a woman with a primary personality disorder: self-defeating, prone to narcissistic injury, and entitled to act out her distress maladaptively. Within this context, her "depression" could seem like a logical extension of, and secondary to, these defects. Treating her depression medically did not eliminate her vulnerability to loss, her protective counterdependent inclinations, or her urges to act upon her distress "badly." However, it helped her greatly with the intensity and frequency of her distress; it helped her gain perspective on "what was life and what was depression"; and it helped her redefine the nature of her "flaw." It was, and is, preferable to her to be treatably depressive than hopelessly self-destructive.

CASE 6: PHILLIP

Phillip entered treatment in the throes of marked depression. He was in his early 30s and single; he had been trained in a profession, but was working as an apprentice long after others would usually strike out on their own. He presented symptomatically with marked depressed mood and agitation; insomnia, anergy, and anhedonia; extreme confusion, indecision, and self-doubt; and frequent despair, hopelessness, and suicidal ideation, based on his conviction that his life was doomed to failure. His periods of depression had begun during his adolescence and had formerly been intermittent, but were occurring with increasing frequency.

At the time of his presentation, Phillip was obsessed with a relationship that was inappropriate and unavailable as a romance. The woman was a friend who clearly saw Phillip as a helpful, supportive "older brother." His preoccupation with her took on many levels of meaning for him, but it especially signified his self-perceived incapacity to have a relationship with a woman, his inability to be successful in anything, and his worthlessness and failure in life. He was paralyzed by obsessional ruminations about all decisions, going into exhaustive detail about the pros and cons of both trivial and important events; he desperately sought direction and reassurance from the therapist.

The younger of two siblings in a close-knit family, Phillip had been a mild-mannered, shy, and cerebral child. He was close to his mother, a housewife, and held his father, a physician, in the highest esteem. He thought he would follow in his father's footsteps, and recalled with affection and admiration going on rounds with his father as a young boy.

When Phillip was 13, his father developed cancer and died several months later after a period of progressive deterioration. Phillip was devastated; he went through adolescence in a fog, and at times was quite depressed. He floundered and muddled his way through school, going off to college only because it was "the thing to do." Without direction, he continued to depend on the guidance of family and friends, who advised him to attend professional school. Throughout his time in school, Phillip read voraciously. Aside from the comfort he found in reading, a part of him felt that if he "cultivated" himself he would be better prepared if and when he ever entered the mainstream of life. His exceptional intellectual abilities carried him through professional school and specialty training, despite his never experiencing any sense of ownership in his career. After completing professional school he took an apprenticeship, where he still remained at the time he sought treatment. He felt trapped in a career not of his making and not of great value in his eyes. He was reluctant either to invest much effort in improving his skills or to go off on his own; he had no confidence in his ability to learn his trade or find another. He was only able to support himself because of a small trust fund.

Phillip had developed a small cadre of good friends, and had continuing close ties with his immediate and extended family. He had cultivated his social skills, and his intellectual and verbal skills enabled him to hide the depth of his despair from others. His relationships with most people were marked by his extreme personal generosity and altruism, an almost complete lack of assertiveness or selfishness, and no hostility. The only aggressive acts in which Phillip could participate were those occurring in the context of intellectual discussions. He could say "no" to no one. He had never dated in high school or college, and his longest relationship had lasted only a few weeks. He had no hope of developing a romantic relationship because of his sense of personal inadequacy and failure, especially because of the paralysis in his work: "Why would anyone want such a mess?"

The formulation that evolved during the early phase of assessment was that Phillip was by temperament and nature a shy, cerebral, unaggressive, and somewhat dependent individual whose development had been distorted by his father's illness and death. His primary source of identification was partially internalized, but the concrete external guide was gone, and whatever self-direction Phillip might have achieved was condemned by his recurrent depression. With his father's death and his mother's recovery and adjustment, Phillip was without objects of rebellion; this further inhibited the development of an assertive and identifiably separate self. Because he lacked a sense of self, and rejected his own sexual or intimate needs as overly aggressive and selfish, his heterosexual development was also stymied. Superimposed upon and further complicating his inhibited and impaired identity, arrested heterosexual development, and paralyzed career development were the recurrent episodes of depression, which served only to create more intense dysfunction and regression. He *was* a mess.

Eschewing medical intervention, Phillip began in psychotherapy three times a week and has continued for 7 years with decreasing frequency. The goals of treatment as they evolved over time included the following:

1. To help Phillip develop insight into the forces that had led him to seek treatment.

2. To reengage him with his work.
3. To help him explore other avenues of personal expression and fulfillment, including a possible career change.
4. To help him develop a satisfying heterosexual relationship.
5. To help him understand the role of depression in his work, relationships, and self-concept, and to treat it pharmacologically if necessary.

It was assumed that as these goals were achieved, Phillip's identity would evolve into one of greater mastery and confidence, and that the identification and exercise of his needs in each of these areas would help him to become more assertive and "self-actualizing." Despite the "mess" of Phllip's life, his therapist developed the conviction that Phillip possessed the capacity to achieve each of these goals. Phillip, through his turmoil and pain, had demonstrated exceptional intellectual and conceptual abilities; an enormous capacity for empathy, compassion, and altruism; wisdom and maturity that were available for others but not himself; an openness and honesty that exposed his humiliation excessively; and a perseverance that belied his suffering.

The earliest phase of treatment involved containing Phillip's extreme turmoil and suicidal preoccupation. He did need concrete guidance to avoid acting upon some of his maladaptive impulses and to encourage him to accept where he was in his career, at least temporarily, so that he could more fully understand the impediments to his work (in addition to depression) and develop sufficient mastery to feel confident that he could apply his skills elsewhere (if he ever decided where that might be). His work inhibition was severe: He would sit for hours unable to attend to a project, his mind wandering off in fantasy or being caught up in his usual vicious cycle—not feeling competent enough to finish a task, and not wanting to invest the effort to become more competent because this would tighten his career trap.

Within a few months, as his depression and turmoil subsided, the dependency of Phillip's desperation evolved into the security of a holding relationship in which the therapist became an idealized, omniscient parent. At one level, the therapist and patient explored and understood this relationship. At another level, Phillip used it as a base of security from which to explore and experiment in the real world, assured that nothing catastrophic would occur and that every risk and accomplishment would be examined.

Phillip began volunteer work with troubled adolescents. He was a natural therapist to whom children gravitated and opened up. He was warm, giving, extremely patient, nonthreatening, and wise; to his surprise, he was also able to be confrontative and to set limits, thus exercising elements of aggression that were new to him. Gradually, he devoted more and more time to this work and began to consider whether he should go to medical school or graduate school to become a psychologist or social worker.

Concurrently, he struggled through his work inhibition and found himself becoming increasingly capable despite his doubts. He eventually opened his own office, then struggled to charge people for his work. Over several years, he has become highly competent at his work; he is sought out because of his knowledge and integrity. As he has become more engaged in his work, his sense of mastery and the satisfaction he has brought to others have helped him appreciate his career, though he continues to undercharge people. His career has become a part of his identity, alongside his continuing involvement with youth.

On the relationship front, Phillip made an effort to become involved with a younger woman whom he met at work. She initially welcomed his interest, but after they became romantically involved, she spurned him. This precipitated a crisis for Phillip in which be persevered in his pursuit of her until her rejection of him was made more openly painful and humiliating. Undaunted, he persisted in his efforts to maintain the relationship at some level; remarkably, he was eventually able to transform a failed romance into a desexualized, supportive friendship.

Subsequently, Phillip struck up a friendship with a woman his age. He and Penny gradually developed a very strong, mutually caring relationship that has tested them both. This relationship has now gone on for several years and recently culminated in marriage. Despite their mutual affection and respect, Phillip and Penny have had considerable difficulties in living together, because of their a very different methods of communication and personal styles. Over the past 3 years, Phillip's individual therapy has been transformed into couple treatment. This reflects the therapist's and patients' understanding that the other goals of treatment have been met.

A year after entering treatment, Phillip had another episode of major depression, which persisted for several weeks. At that time, the depression was primarily affecting Phillip's work because of insomnia, anergy, and cognitive impairment. With pressure from his therapist, he consented to antidepressant treatment and was placed on desipramine. He responded well, with some anticholinergic side effects, and continued on the drug for several months. He has had two subsequent recurrences, each treated effectively with fluoxetine; he has been on fluoxetine continuously for the past 2 years. Despite this, he has had several brief periods of 1–2 days when he experiences acute fatigue, anergy, anhedonia, irritability, and cognitive impairment. When these episodes occur, he fights through them to complete his work, often hides his feelings from Penny, and generally treats them as a nuisance to be tolerated until they pass. They do not escalate into the all-encompassing, hopeless, self-deprecating, suicidal states that he experienced prior to treatment. Depression no longer represents a threat to Phillip's self-esteem or life, his career choice, or his relationship. Although he may be more irritable, may be less patient, or may feel more entitled within his relationship with Penny at these times, he is usually able to recognize this and contain it.

The relationship between Phillip and his therapist has also evolved. In the early stages of powerful positive transference, the therapist was quite reluctant to express many opinions other than those that were essential for Phillip's survival and functioning. An exception to this was, and has continued to be, the therapist's genuine appreciation and admiration for qualities that Phillip could not appreciate in himself or that were undermined by his depression.

As treatment went on, Phillip could gradually relinquish his insistence on reassurance from the therapist. He subsequently developed a stronger sense of his own qualities and strengths, and eventually ventured to criticize his therapist or to ignore him at times. With the gradual rehumanizing of the therapist, the indications for more intense, "reconstructive" treatment have subsided; were it not for the current couple work, ongoing psychotherapy would be of a very limited nature, incorporating the monitoring of his antidepressant treatment.

Phillip's case provides an example of depression as a force that can alter development. Personality structures can become fixed, not simply state-dependent qualities that are reversible with control of the depression. Phillip's premorbid inclinations, the death of his father, and his subsequent depression conspired to disrupt his development in numerous ways. Each facet of personality difficulty had to be addressed separately from the depression, as well as in conjunction with it. Correcting developmental disturbances does not alter people's vulnerability to depression, but enables them to deal with it more effectively and with fewer consequences for their lives.

The initial psychotherapeutic efforts focused on opening Phillip's opportunities for the development of career, relationships, and self-esteem—all of which had been stymied by long-standing depression. Definitive medical control of his depression enabled Phillip to obtain reinforcement for these gains, and also prevented them from being subverted by the forces of depression.

FINAL COMMENTS

As we have noted at the beginning of the chapter, the cases described here illustrate variations on the basic themes of treatment. In every patient a therapist sees, there is a complex interaction of depression with personality. The treatment of depression can help the patient and therapist sort out the nature of this interaction and assess the residual problems once depression is controlled. At times, there are no residual problems and there is little work to do. At other times, the problems become focused on sustaining the treatment of depression, and psychotherapy evolves into working with "resistance." Finally, in cases where depression has been long-standing and has distorted developmental processes, considerable psychotherapeutic work may be required to help in the "re-development" of personality.

The biological perspective presented in this book provides a framework for understanding this interaction. The creativity of clinicians will yield many different variations as they apply their craft to such an orientation.

·9·

Applications to Other Clinical Disorders and States

Biologically informed psychotherapy has been described thus far in its application to the treatment of depression (i.e., BIPD). Its principles are easily extended to other major psychiatric disorders or states, even though their specific applications will be different, depending upon the idiosyncrasies of a given condition. The fundamental principles that can be applied to other disorders or states are as follows:

1. The condition has core features that are biological and autonomous.
2. The "language" of the condition is well defined, but is often misattributed.
3. The regression associated with the expression of the illness must be understood and not misinterpreted.
4. The condition has no cure; its expression may be controlled medically, but the vulnerability to it will persist.
5. Education and coping with the condition give the victim the best chances of control over the process.
6. Accepting the illness and its nature is critical for limiting the possible devastation that can occur.

In this chapter, we briefly review a number of other disorders or states to which these principles may apply: various anxiety disorders, schizophrenia, and manic or hypomanic states. We conclude with some comments on the third principle in particular (i.e., the understanding and management of regression).

189

ANXIETY DISORDERS

Panic Disorder and Related Conditions

Many believe that the core disturbance in panic disorder is spontaneous and inappropriate firing of the autonomic fight-or-flight mechanism, located in the locus coeruleus and the adrenal medullary system (Klein, 1964, 1981; Sheehan, 1983). This "hairtrigger" discharge of the mechanism, when misinterpreted as a warning of danger rather than as a random and meaningless physiological event, can lead to secondary and tertiary psychological phenomena that become the true morbidity associated with the disorder.

A panic attack itself is one of the more disquieting and potentially frightening experiences that many people will have in their lives. If it occurs in the context of immediate psychological events that are "understandable" or that represent an actual but not life-threatening danger (e.g., while one is studying for an exam or before one makes a speech), it will probably be attributed to those circumstances, and a further search for meaning will be unnecessary. However, when panic attacks occur in clusters, these states often precipitate an escalating catastrophic attribution, even in cases where the individual may identify a general context of stress. Because they often occur "out of the blue" and present a myriad of physical and psychological symptoms of intense anxiety, those who suffer from panic disorder will frequently believe that they are dying, having a heart attack, losing control and acting out, or going crazy (Sheehan, 1983).

The consequences of such recurrent states may include the development of even more significant psychopathological responses. First, the individual develops a dread of recurrence of the anxiety and becomes hypervigilant—a condition known as "anticipatory anxiety." When left unchecked and untreated, this anxiety can spread and become generalized. It also frequently develops autonomy; that is, it becomes dissociated from its initial precipitant (the panic states) and evolves into a chronic state, which causes considerable suffering and dysfunction and is difficult to treat (Sheehan, 1983). Generalized anxiety can be understood as the equivalent of the autonomic hyperarousal associated with posttraumatic stress disorder (McNally & Lukach, 1992). In this instance, the trauma is the recurrent panic attack.

Another pathological response to recurrent panic states is the development of phobic avoidance (Sheehan, 1983). The individual attributes the occurrence of panic attacks to a set of circumstances that may or may not be directly associated with the attacks, and develops a specific fear of those circumstances. The feared circumstances may be seen as the causes of the panic (e.g., heights, bridges, open spaces), or may be seen as things to avoid lest panic should occur and escape should be necessary (e.g., theaters, elevators). The fear of embarrassment or humiliation over what the fearful individuals believe others might see or what they themselves might do will often lead to a more general avoidance of people.

Effective treatment of the components of panic disorder, as well as of generalized anxiety and the different types of phobic avoidance, has been accomplished with a variety of psychopharmacological (Klein, 1964; Klein et al., 1985; Ballenger et al., 1988; Fyer & Samberg, 1988) and cognitive-behavioral (Barlow, 1988; Alford et al., 1990; Clark, 1988) approaches. As has been the case for all symptomatic disorders and states, psychodynamically oriented psychotherapists have understood all of these symptoms as manifestations of unresolved psychological conflict that require exploration, uncovering, and working through as the means of resolution. By contrast, an integrative approach to these conditions using the principles of biologically informed psychotherapy incorporates elements of treatment that have already demonstrated efficacy for depression.

Education

Patients with panic disorder and related conditions learn that panic attacks are normal physiological events that have gone awry. Vulnerability to such events is genetically inheritable, and a "no-fault" attitude should be taken toward their occurrence. A panic attack is not a manifestation of personal weakness; it does not mean that one cannot handle life's stresses. The panic event itself is "meaningless" and should not be misinterpreted as (1) a psychological manifestation of unresolved conflicts, (2) a warning of an impending heart attack, or (3) the first sign of losing control and becoming violent or self-destructive. Education serves to decatastrophize the event and actually to "trivialize" it. In this process of "trivialization," patients must be made aware of the absence of danger in such occurrences. Although they may feel terrible, they are not unsafe; nothing serious will happen to them. Finally, the education of patients should include, as necessary, an understanding of how panic states can lead to both generalized anxiety and the formation of phobias.

The language of these conditions is the anxiety itself, which, when misinterpreted, tells people to avoid many things besides the specific situations or circumstances in which panic attacks occur. Many people believe that their bodies are telling them to take it easy, avoid stress, change relationships, or quit jobs, because the contexts in which symptoms are manifested always include the "universal conflicts of life" in relationships, work, and self-concepts. The regressions that are inevitable consequences of such symptomatic expressions will often push people toward "simplifying their lives"; unfortunately, this nearly always involves extricating themselves from the complexities that give life richness and meaning. Anxiety will always press in the direction of avoidance. Treatments should be counterphobic and counteravoidant.

Psychodynamic Exploration

Psychodynamic exploration will be useful in different ways. A knowledge of a particular patient's dynamics will anticipate the areas of psychological vulnerability to which the patient is likely to attribute the symptoms. A preemptive observation of such a likelihood may be very useful in helping the patient appreciate the sequence of events. The invariable experience of loss of control can be countered by the authoritative reassurance that this state is a product of the panic and will subside. The concurrence of life events whose meaning is significant to the context of the patient's anxiety can be explored as a contributing factor without being defined as "causal." Finally, any forms of regression that ensue can be examined as temporary consequences of the anxiety and not as indications of lifelong inadequacy.

Coping Skills Exploration, Training, and Support

Coping skills to counteract the impact of panic disorder and related conditions draw upon specific techniques that are frequently applied in the cognitive-behavioral treatment of anxiety disorders: relaxation training; guided imagery; and deliberate exposure and hierarchical desensitization for phobic symptoms.

Work with Significant Others

Therapeutic work with a spouse or family proceeds in a fashion similar to that described in Chapter 5 for the treatment of depression. Anxiety symptoms are not likely to insinuate themselves within the personality as pervasively as depressive symptoms, so the nature of the disturbances within a family system will look different. The avoidance and inhibition caused by the fear of panic attacks are the more usual sources of disturbances. These may lead to regressions that affect relationships, or to a constriction of activities and travel, a fear of novelty, and a general dampening of the richness of life. With panic disorder and related conditions, there is seldom a need for significant others as monitors; the symptoms are inherently discomforting and identifiable, and those who suffer from them will want to seek help.

Case Example 1

Robert, a 30-year-old physician, came to treatment in a state of marked insomnia and agitation; he felt he was "falling apart," and feared that this state of mind would persist indefinitely. He felt sufficiently "out of control" that he was concerned that he could commit suicide, even though he had no suicidal impulses and certainly wanted to live. He described having had several panic attacks per week over the previous month. These emerged from a context of several stressors: uncertainty about his career; an acute career disappointment with marked narcissistic injury; financial difficulties; and the approach of his board examinations.

Robert had been in an automobile accident a year earlier. A tire blew out while he was driving on the freeway. His car spun out of control, crashed into a guard rail, and stopped in the far left lane facing oncoming traffic. He received only minor injuries, but he developed anxiety about driving and experienced several panic attacks during the following months, with symptoms of anxiety, palpitations, shortness of breath, sweating, and dread. He persisted (out of necessity) in his driving and was able to overcome much of the anxiety of doing so, but he continued to avoid that particular stretch of road. Furthermore, his previous love of driving was gone.

Prior to this incident, Robert had experienced a single episode of panic 4 years earlier, but had had several episodes of pavor nocturnus (panic attacks that awaken one during non-REM sleep). His health had been otherwise excellent. He did not drink, smoke, or use drugs or caffeine.

Robert's developmental and social history were unremarkable. He had enjoyed a nontraumatic and stable family life, constant academic and social success, and uninterrupted career development. His 6-year marriage had had early financial and adjustment struggles, but was currently a solid and committed relationship, disturbed now only by his turmoil.

At the time of Robert's presentation, he was diagnosed with a panic disorder. His previous series of recurrent panic attacks had resolved without treatment. However, the greatest risk to Robert, who had always viewed himself as confident and quite accomplished, was his perception that his recent series of events marked the beginning of an inexorable decline. His view of his immediate experience was catastrophic: He was "out of control," anxious, and sleep-deprived. Though he was not yet impaired in his work, he anticipated that this was next.

The therapist's first intervention was to convey to Robert that what Robert was experiencing was definable, very common, almost stereotypical, and (despite his fears) usually easily manageable. Panic disorder and its consequences were discussed phenomenologically and, because Robert was a physician, with a highly specific scientific focus. The therapist suggested that Robert had a long-standing (though usually unexpressed) vulnerability to panic, which until now had had minimal consequences. The occurrence of anxiety symptoms following his auto accident had been accepted as a normal reaction, and Robert had had little elaboration of the primary symptoms of anxiety (though his limited avoidance had persisted). When anxiety symptoms later emerged without a clear precipitant (even with background stressors that may or may not have been relevant), Robert began to attribute his evolving symptoms to his lack of ability to cope with the issues in his life, and to generalize this supposed inadequacy to every phase of his life. His concept of himself as an autonomous, capable, and generative person was changing. Perhaps he had been living with an illusion, and this state was the "true" one— the one that would persist. This view was quite demoralizing.

Despite Robert's distress, he was *not* suicidal in any clinical sense. It was important to convey to him that his fears about suicide reflected a normal variant of the experience of being out of control that patients with panic often have: "If I am out of control, I could do anything." The therapist assured him that this would not occur. He offered a "written guarantee," which was deemed unnecessary. This offer was made in the context of the therapist's awareness that a good alliance had already been established in their first session, and that Robert's nature was methodical, rational, and not impulsive; it was specifically directed at an already evolving strategy of trivializing the meaning of his symptoms (not his suffering). To underscore the limited contribution of Robert's stressors to his syndrome, the therapist explored previous periods of even greater stress in his life that he had handled naturally, without dysfunction or symptoms. Robert agreed that his vulnerability to panic had been greater following his accident, and that his current stressors, though inherently upsetting, did not account for the intensity of his response.

Robert was treated with a low dose of an antidepressant (imipramine, 50 mg) at night to help him sleep and to abort his panic symptoms. He was encouraged to drive on the "unsafe" strip of highway; to adopt an attitude toward his symptoms that "It's only anxiety"; and to tolerate his discomfort as best as he could without ascribing any particular meaning to it. Robert was seen on six occasions over a 6-month period. He had occasional episodes of panic, but following his first session, he was able to treat subsequent episodes as uncomfortable nuisances. His general anxiety dissolved quickly; his phobia about the "unsafe" road was gone within a month as he went out of his way to challenge himself. After 3 months, he discontinued his medication without concern about subsequent recurrences. At an 18-month follow-up, he was doing well.

It is likely that Robert will experience panic symptoms again in the future, either spontaneously or in the context of life stressors. However, given his understanding of panic disorder, his counterphobic strivings for mastery, and his healthy adaptive skills, it is highly unlikely that such a recurrence will disrupt his life. If symptoms become the source of too great or too frequent discomfort, they can be controlled easily enough with antidepressant or anxiolytic medications.

Case Example 2

Ten years ago, John, a faculty physician in his mid-30s, sought treatment for panic disorder. During the prior 4 weeks, he had been experiencing multiple spontaneous panic attacks daily; these included symptoms of overwhelming dread, tachycardia, queasiness, and dyspnea. His anxiety quickly generalized and was at a constant, high level. He feared losing control, and had images of hurting himself or killing his wife and three children. He became increasingly phobic about leaving home and driving his car, and even took some time off work. History revealed that John had had episodes of panic attacks for brief periods earlier in his life. These had resolved without sequelae.

Shortly after his panic attacks began, John consulted a psychoanalyst who evaluated him, sent him for psychological testing, and gave him a small amount of alprazolam, which helped his anxiety. He was referred to a medical school faculty psychiatrist (because of his insurance), with the suggestion that he has "a lot of issues with his father and with being in control." He thus came for treatment with a "prescription" for intensive, long-term psychotherapy. The psychoanalyst's report posited that the sources of his symptoms included fatigue, pressure to perform, and a "fear of imitating his patients and losing control over himself" (which would cause him great embarrassment and humiliation if it occurred at work). All of these factors were seen as having their roots in earlier fears and childhood anxieties. Dynamic issues were identified: "a deep-seated longing to be rewarded with love, attention, support, and total acceptance"; fears of abandonment; striving for mastery as compensation against his helplessness in the face of a childhood illness; and an inclination toward martyrdom. "He is eager for relief from his agonizing state and ready now to accept the fact he is suffering an emotional as opposed to an organic or physical problem. The danger with this man is relieving his symptoms without taking him further down the road of self-understanding."

At that point, John's contact with the psychoanalyst had thoroughly convinced him that he was "totally fucked up" and needed a "psychological exorcism." His psychological regression was understood by the analyst as a manifestation of substantial psychopathology lying dormant in his personality structure. John's vulnerability made him more likely to accept any authoritative view of his ailment, and he was prepared to follow through with this prescription, despite some reservations. These reservations stemmed from two sources.

First and foremost, although John felt horribly impaired at that point in time, he had always thought of himself as "a pretty healthy guy." He was under some stresses: pressure to publish, the life of a clinician, the anticipation of assuming greater responsibility for his aging parents. On the other hand, he had alway been a bit overextended; he enjoyed the challenges of clinical pressure and of bearing responsibility. He had a strong and close marriage to a woman who was his best friend and support. He was actively and intimately involved in his children's development. He was a leader in his church and had an active social life. He loved his work, had an excellent reputation as a clinician and teacher, and maintained good relationships with his colleagues. Furthermore, John had excellent insight into the major dynamic issues that had been identified.

John's other reservation about wholesale acceptance of the analyst's "prescription" was that as a physician who encountered patients with anxiety disorders quite often, he was aware of a good deal of the research literature on anxiety disorders and their biological underpinnings. He found this view appealing, but felt uncomfortable because it "let him off the hook" too easily.

The medical school faculty therapist took the following biologically informed stance: John did indeed seem to be a psychologically healthy and strong person. All of the elements of his regression were fully understandable as manifestations of his panic disorder—a disorder that he seemed to have had in mild and infrequent form throughout his adult life. It would be important to control his symptoms and help him resume functioning. (John had not understood why, when he seemed barely able to walk from his car to the office, the analyst was so concerned about his relationship with his mother.) Once that was accomplished, he would be in a better position to assess how "screwed up" he might be psychologically.

After a week on an adequate dose of alprazolam, John's anxiety symptoms subsided. His panic symptoms did not return, though mild symptoms of generalized anxiety did persist, diminishing over time but never disappearing fully. It was as if his "rheostat" for anxiety had been turned up slightly. This residual anxiety could be controlled with small amounts of alprazolam (0.125 mg twice a day), but it persisted.

John's life was quickly back in order. He tried every personal experiment that he and his therapist could concoct to see whether he could discontinue the alprazolam and still feel comfortable. He incorporated relaxation training, exercise, prayer and meditation, and cognitive and educational elements into his regimen. He went for months without medication to prove that he could function fully with the anxiety, and did so. Periodically, however, he would decide to reinstitute the alprazolam: "Should I be uncomfortable just to prove a point?" In his ever less frequent (weekly, then monthly, then quarterly, then yearly) meetings with his psychiatrist, he would deliberate over the never-ending dilemma: "The analogy to requiring insulin if you're diabetic works for a long time. Then I wonder if I can go without the Xanax." His conflict over this dependency has not been fully resolved (nor is it likely ever to be resolved). Ten years later, John is living an effective and fulfilling life with a minuscule amount of alprazolam daily. He had a panic attack "out of the blue" a couple years ago. "It was strange to observe it happening in me. It was uncomfortable, but that's all." He was amazed by the contrast of that event and his detached reaction to it with his debilitating presentation at the start of treatment.

John was a person who came to the treatment setting with excellent internal resources: intelligence, insight, education about anxiety, strong interpersonal skills, capacities to cope adaptively, and an excellent support network. All that he needed from treatment were effective pharmacological management and "protection" from misattribution of his symptoms. Usually such misattribution proceeds from a patient's interpretation of his or her symptoms, and there certainly was some of that in John's case (which cleared quickly with treatment).

However, had John followed the psychoanalyst's recommendation, he might have spent an indefinite period of time (because some symptoms did persist) and money on treatment, and might have faced enormous potential morbidity (secondary to the evolving phobic avoidance and work disability). Furthermore, the process of dynamic psychotherapy would have confirmed his regressive views of his fundamental inadequacy, neuroticism, and maladaptiveness, whether he got better or not. Failure to improve would have been attributed to resistance or secondary gain—further proof of his inadequacy. Improvement would confirm the assessment, at least until the next exacerbation of the disorder.

Biologically informed psychotherapy does not posit pathology in character, but in the physical body. John's "personal failure" or "weakness of character" did not cause him to have severe anxiety symptoms. Furthermore, patients with moderate to severe symptomatology must exert enormous energy and determination to persist in their functioning. They should be lauded for their efforts, rather than chastised for limitations created by their illness.

Obsessive–Compulsive Disorder

Until the demonstration of the effectiveness of the serotonergic agent clomipramine (and subsequently of the SSRIs) in treating obsessive–compulsive disorder (OCD) (Goodman et al., 1992), this disorder had the potential to create enormous suffering and disruption of normal functioning, without much hope from treatment. Patients with severe OCD were subjected to every psychological, behavioral, and somatic treatment available, with limited results (Hollander et al., 1988). Many eventually had neurosurgical ablative procedures performed (with some benefit) to reduce their suffering. Currently, the combination of serotonergic antidepressant medications with behavioral treatments (primarily techniques of exposure and response prevention) has proven effective in treating most forms of OCD (Schwartz et al., 1992; Baxter et al., 1992).

OCD also lends itself well to other principles of biologically informed psychotherapy. Because the symptoms of OCD are so stereotypical, only the most "die-hard" dynamic therapist will attribute meaning to these symptoms. A team at UCLA (Schwartz et al., 1992) has developed a manual for cognitive-biobehavioral self-treatment for OCD, which teaches the patient to appreciate OCD symptoms as artifacts of brain disturbances rather than as meaningful messages (obsessions) that require behavioral responses (compulsions). This perspective contributes to the patient's ability to adhere to the program of response prevention. This method has been so effective that it has been shown (by means of functional brain imaging techniques) to reverse the hypermetabolism associated with areas of the brain (e.g., the caudate nucleus) that are activated by OCD (Baxter et al., 1992).

SCHIZOPHRENIA

Until the 1960s, a substantial proportion of the mental health community viewed schizophrenia as a primary psychological disorder—the product of developmental disturbances, including the "schizophrenogenic mother" (Weiner, 1975). Even as antipsychotic medications began to be incorporated into the treatment of most psychotic patients, there remained a strong bias toward uncovering what was "really wrong" with the patient and a tendency to interpret psychotic processes as manifestations of core conflicts that were central to the disorder. Although this view still has some staunch adherents, the majority of mental health practitioners have come to view schizophrenia as a severe brain disorder whose symptoms have no more meaning than the weakness associated with muscular dystrophy.

This recognition that hallucinations, delusions, and negative symptoms are simply products of brain functions gone awry has enabled clinicians treating schizophrenia to employ many of the principles of BIPD as described in this book. Indeed, these principles have been more readily applied to treating schizophrenic patients than depressed patients, in part because schizophrenia has been easier than depression to accept as an illness. At another level, clinicians are also less likely to misinterpret the language of the disorder, even though patients may experience a powerful moral imperative to act upon such manifestations as their ideas of reference, command hallucinations, and delusions. Therapists may be unable to convince patients that their symptoms are merely the "illness talking." However, often patients can learn this and may preserve sufficient observing ego and capacity for distancing themselves from their symptoms. Even when patients are "captured" by their illness, therapists know that they are ill and that their illness can probably be controlled with antipsychotic medication.

In the treatment of schizophrenia, and more recently in that of depression, there has been a growing recognition that for most patients the disorder is a chronic or recurring illness that waxes and wanes, requiring continual monitoring, education, and family involvement (Fava & Kaji, 1994; Hogarty et al., 1986). Psychotherapy is aimed at helping patients cope as best as possible with their lifelong illness and its effects on their lives. In other words, psychotherapy for schizophrenia is to a great extent already biologically informed.

MANIC OR HYPOMANIC STATES

Inasmuch as manic or hypomanic episodes are almost invariably associated with depressive episodes, it is understandable that any psychotherapy addressing the problems of depression will be part of the manic or hypomanic patient's treatment and will incorporate all of the elements of BIPD. Manic and hypomanic states, however, have unique characteristics that require some modifications of BIPD.

Central to such modifications is the recognition of the *power* of these states. A patient experiencing an intense manic episode will exhibit boundless energy, grandiosity, fearless impulsivity, and driven (though often distractible) goal seeking. Usually in both manic and hypomanic states, patients are "captured" by the altered states more powerfully and more completely than in depressive states of equivalent severity. Moreover, the language of manic and hypomanic states is often ego-syntonic; that is, the sense of well-being (or even the irritability) is experienced as real, genuine, and appropriate. It is subjected neither to personal scrutiny nor to a therapist's influence, criticism, or even examination. Unlike depressive states, which are inherently painful, hypomanic and manic states result in no wish for relief. Finally, in contrast to patients with depression (who may be passive or paralyzed and amenable to direction by a firm therapist), patients with mania or hypomania are almost invariably "running the show." There are some exceptions—usually patients who are hypomanic, well educated about their illness, well allied with their therapists, and not captured by the disordered state. However, the usual inaccessibility of manic and hypomanic patients dictates the following modifications in their treatment.

First, education must take place during periods of mood stability. Patients who are euthymic or even moderately depressed can appreciate the risks that hypomanic or manic states pose to their health (because of substance use or sexual promiscuity), their finances (because of reckless spending or risky business decisions), or their relationships (because of grandiosity, irritability, or impulsivity). Under these circumstances, they can understand the course and language of mania or hypomania and the need to seek help and control it at its first appearance.

A second consequence of these rapidly evolving and powerful states is that the monitoring function of significant others becomes much more crucial—both to help a patient recognize changes in mood as they are occurring, and to inform the therapist when the patient is disinclined or unable to do so. Having a network of family, friends, and even enlightened colleagues at work may mean the difference between rapid intervention and prolonged disability. One note of caution: The best-laid plans often go astray. Despite the best efforts of therapist, patient, and significant others, it is in the nature of mania or hypomania that when it occurs, others may not be able to influence its course.

Finally, because of the potentially destructive power of mania and hypomania, a clinician and patient may have fewer optionss and less flexibility in regard to medication treatment and prophylaxis. In a case where the power of the patient's state has made it difficult or impossible to contain it whenever it occurs, the need for maintenance/prophylactic pharmacotherapy becomes essential.

COMMENTS ON UNDERSTANDING AND MANAGING REGRESSION

Throughout our discussions of the treatment of depression and other disorders, we have acknowledged the ubiquity of regressive states. Regression is a universal product of illness, both in psychiatric and in other medical disorders. The language of regression is often misinterpreted by patients. They tend to interpret their immediate perceptions of inade-quacy, dependency, or weakness not as the normal, state-dependent consequences of pain, suffering, and disability, but as stable reflections of their personality flaws and as messages that they should be coping more effectively with their life circumstances. Viewing such regressions in the context of depression, BIPD maintains that exploration and active ef-forts to counter such misattributions will both preserve patients' self-esteem and prevent them from acting upon their distorted perceptions.

This same principle can be applied both to regressions resulting from other psychiatric disorders and states, and to these occurring outside the context of psychiatric illness. Clinicians frequently see people who are in the throes of turmoil and whose acute regressive states belie the fact that they are fundamentally healthy. Both clinicians and patients can get caught up in the specifics of such states and can overpathologize them in a detrimental way. The following case example of a woman with an adjustment disorder is used to illustrate this possibility.

Christine, a 32-year-old businesswoman, married to Joe for the past 6 years, came for evaluation a week after Joe announced he was leaving her to be with a woman with whom he had been involved before their marriage. Christine felt as if her "world was caving in." During the past week, she had not slept well, couldn't eat, was crying easily, and was making mistakes at work. Up to now, she had never been sick or missed work; she had prided herself on her self-sufficiency and her generally positive outlook on life. She had never spoken with a therapist because she had "never felt the need."

Since Joe's announcement, Christine had been preoccupied with her feelings of anger, abandonment, and betrayal toward Joe. However, she also ruminated over her undesirability, dependency, and inadequacy in both her relationships and her work. She began to regret her choice to pursue a career, and to wonder whether she shouldn't have stayed at home and had children to cement their marital relationship. She feared she would never have another relationship with a man and would never have children. She believed that she had made a wreck of her life, even though she could see Joe's contributions to her current distress.

This example is almost stereotypical, not only in its depiction of an all-too-common set of circumstances, but also in the nature of Chris-tine's responses to her situation. Christine was at a point of substantial vulnerability—both to those regressive forces that were undermining her functioning and self-concept, and to the potential influence of a therapist's interpretation of her experiences. Left to her own devices, Christine would probably recover from this regressed state. Over a brief period of time, her anger at Joe would be likely to crystallize. She would probably assume some appropriate level of personal responsibility for the failure of their relationship, and would probably return to the state of confidence and competence that had characterized her before Joe's announcement. If this did not happen, there would be a high index of suspicion that a depressive illness was evolving.

A therapist who did not recognize the language of regression or understand the time-limited, state-dependent nature of Christine's experience, or who placed a high premium on the heuristic value of regression, might intervene by encouraging the deepening of the regression. In Christine's state of emotional and cognitive fluidity, such an approach might reinforce her ego-dystonic perceptions and might further undermine her sense of self.

We encourage clinicians to approach this type of situation-specific regression in the same way as we have recommended approaching it in BIPD: as a time-limited, state-dependent series of distorted perceptions that can be understood in both idiosyncratic (personal development) and universal (stereotypic) ways. A biologically informed therapist would support Christine's view of herself at her most adaptive, despite the recognition that her regressed state had some reality basis, which the stress of her current situation had exaggerated and distorted. An example of such an intervention might be as follows:

THERAPIST: Your distress is understandable, and you may want to talk about it some more. On the other hand, there's no way to avoid feeling awful for a while. It is my impression that you're able to tolerate the way you feel without any significant consequences to your health, your relationship, your job, or your life. I'm actually more concerned about how you are interpreting some of your thoughts and feelings. This crisis has left you questioning a number of long-standing issues with which you seemed to have come to terms before now. It's hard to know what, if any, significance these doubts and concerns have when you feel so bad. See if you can suspend your judgment about these until some of this turmoil has passed.

The purposes of an intervention such as this are several. First, it defines the suffering as normal and unavoidable. In addition, the therapist's statement of confidence in the patient's capacity to cope with this turmoil without risk (based on an assessment of the fundamental "health" of the patient's personality) shores up those doubts and fears that are stirred up by the emerging regressive attributions of dependency, undesirability, or the like. These doubts and fears are further undermined by the therapist's identifying them as predictable and normal consequences of such turmoil. The door is left open for the therapist and patient to examine these issues further, but the patient's strength and ability are confirmed by making such contact optional and noting that it may not be necessary. "Flight into health" is desirable.

In Christine's case, the fact of her regression was not *prima facie* evidence of personality disturbance. Unless there was other evidence of such disturbance, the first therapeutic task would be the prevention of misattribution and worsening of her normal regression. This would not preclude the possibility that Christine and her therapist might choose to examine any of the previously described "issues" in the future. In contrast to traditional approaches, however, such an examination should strike "when the iron is cold," so both therapist and patient can appreciate that the "issue" is clinically significant.

Although this example does not illustrate the application of BIPD to an illness, it demonstrates how one specific element of BIPD can be utilized in many different circumstances where regression occurs— not only in psychiatric illnesses, but in all of life's crises, and in medical illnesses affecting either oneself or loved ones.